# Physical development

**Planning and Assessment** **Stepping Stones** **Early Learning Goals** **Practical activity ideas**

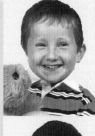
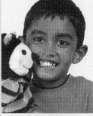
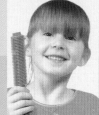
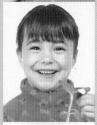
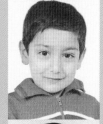
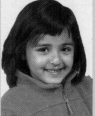

**Jean Evans**

**British Library Cataloguing-in-Publication Data** A catalogue record for this book is available from the British Library.

**ISBN 0 439 98354 1**

# Author
Jean Evans

**Editor**
Lesley Sudlow

**Designer**
Heather C Sanneh

**Assistant Editor**
Saveria Mezzana

**Illustrations**
Mary Hall

**Series Designer**
Clare Brewer

**Cover photography**
Derek Cooknell

**Text © 2003 Jean Evans**
**© 2003 Scholastic Ltd**

Designed using Adobe Pagemaker

Published by Scholastic Ltd,
Villiers House,
Clarendon Avenue,
Leamington Spa,
Warwickshire CV32 5PR

Visit our website at www.scholastic.co.uk
Printed by Proost NV, Belgium

1 2 3 4 5 6 7 8 9 0    3 4 5 6 7 8 9 0 1 2

**Acknowledgements**
Qualifications and Curriculum Authority for the use of extracts from the QCA/DfEE document *Curriculum Guidance for the Foundation Stage* © 2000 Qualifications and Curriculum Authority.
Every effort has been made to trace copyright holders and the publishers apologise for any inadvertent omissions.

**Physical development**

# Contents

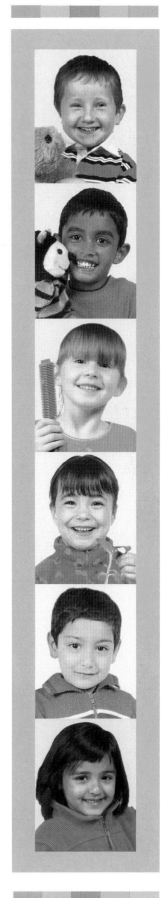

**Physical development**

**Physical development**

# Introduction

This series of six books provides professionals working in nurseries, pre-schools, playgroups and Reception classes, as well as childminders in home settings, with clear guidance about how to plan, deliver and assess a high-quality early years curriculum for three- to five-year-olds. In this book you will find a wealth of stimulating and practical play activities to cover the Early Learning Goals, identified by the Qualifications and Curriculum Authority (QCA) as set out in detail in the document *Curriculum Guidance for the Foundation Stage,* and the Stepping Stones leading to those Goals. The ideas suggested can be applied equally well to the documents on pre-school education published for Scotland, Wales and Northern Ireland.

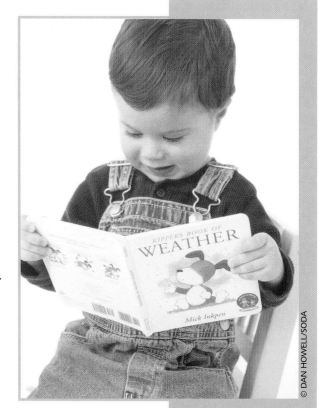

Pages 9 to 14 of this book consider in detail the importance of planning for progression throughout the Foundation Stage and explain the significance of long-, medium- and short-term planning for Physical development. In addition, planning for equal opportunities, including catering for the specific requirements of children with special educational needs (SEN), or children from different ethnic groups, is discussed. Advice is given on organisation of staff and setting up a suitable play environment to extend learning opportunities for Physical development.

Pages 15 to 18 of this book consider the relevance of assessment and recommend different methods of assessment. Advice is given on gathering evidence of the children's developing knowledge, skills and attitudes through the Stepping Stones.

## The importance of physical development
Between the ages of three and five, children are making rapid strides towards independence. By the end of this time, most children will have started school and will be learning to cope with a busy day full of exciting new physical challenges. Encouraging children to exercise and develop good co-ordination in their early years will help them to approach this new phase of their lives with confidence. As they take part in regular exercise and vigorous activities, they will associate physical exertion with enjoyment. They will develop stamina and a positive approach to fitness that will continue in subsequent years, and every new skill that they master will increase their confidence and self-esteem.

## Physical development in the Foundation Stage
The document *Curriculum Guidance for the Foundation Stage* (QCA) states, 'Effective physical development helps children develop a positive

# Introduction

sense of well-being'. Physical development within the Foundation Stage focuses on developing children's control, co-ordination, movement and manipulative skills. In addition, it encourages them to become confident about their physical abilities and raises their awareness of the importance of a healthy lifestyle. Those involved in the care and education of children within the Foundation Stage should ensure that children are given opportunities to develop these skills and attitudes.

The role of the early years practitioner in promoting children's physical development includes:

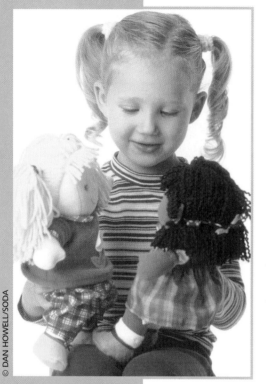

© DAN HOWELL/SODA

- providing children with stimulating and exciting physical activities both indoors and outdoors
- ensuring that children have a safe space to work in, both indoors and outdoors, and that they are dressed appropriately for each activity
- encouraging children to take time to explore and adapt their movements in the light of their experiences
- introducing children to a wide range of interesting experiences to which they can respond through movement
- providing a good selection of interesting items to handle in order to develop small movement skills
- introducing children to the language of movement and to words of instruction associated with actions
- encouraging children to move safely on apparatus and when handling large objects
- ensuring that children with physical disabilities have the time and opportunity to develop their physical skills, and appropriate professional support to do so
- providing extra adult support for individual children, if necessary, to enable them to achieve greater physical independence.

## How to use this book

This book recognises the importance of children's physical development, and the activities within it promote the early recognition of this by giving ideas to encourage children to develop new physical skills and appreciate the need for a good diet and healthy lifestyle. The activities can be used independently or included in topics such as 'Growing', 'All about me' and 'My body'. Suggestions are given throughout the book for raising children's awareness of safety issues and encouraging them to handle equipment correctly.

## Aspects of learning

Each of the six Areas of Learning within the Foundation Stage is divided into separate aspects of learning, and these aspects, or clusters, are further subdivided into relevant Early Learning Goals, as set out in the *Curriculum Guidance for the Foundation Stage*. There are five aspects of learning of Early Learning Goals for Physical development. They are:

- Movement – Move with confidence, imagination and in safety; move with control and co-ordination; travel around, under, over and through balancing and climbing equipment.

■ Sense of space – Show awareness of space, of themselves and of others.
■ Health and bodily awareness – Recognise the importance of keeping healthy and those things which contribute to this; recognise the changes that happen to their bodies when they are active.
■ Using equipment – Use a range of small and large equipment.
■ Using tools and materials – Handle tools, objects, construction and malleable materials safely and with increasing control.

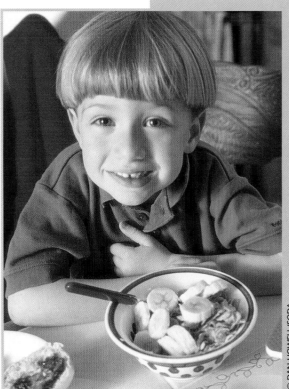

© DAN HOWELL/SODA

## Progression through the Foundation Stage
It is important to realise that children will not master the physical skills referred to in this book all at the same age, and that there will be a wide difference in their abilities at any given time. Each activity chapter within this book focuses on a different aspect of learning, and the practical ideas given cover all the Early Learning Goals and the Stepping Stones. A Stepping Stone is included for each activity, so that it is possible to plan for the children to work at their own pace, building gradually upon their existing skills, knowledge and attitudes, in small but significant steps. The Stepping Stones are colour-coded to show whether the activity is at the simplest level (yellow), at a higher level (blue) or at the highest level (green), to match the colours used to show progression in the document *Curriculum Guidance for the Foundation Stage.*

## The activity pages
There are 12 activity ideas in each chapter, all following the same format. Each activity aims to encourage the children to work towards a specific Early Learning Goal and is designed to promote a definite Stepping Stone. Advice is given regarding the size of the group, but this is flexible according to the size of your setting, number of staff and needs of individual children. Resources required for the activity are also listed, as well as suggested timing, but again these are flexible and can be adapted if necessary. The 'Preparation' section indicates any prior organisation that is needed, while the 'What to do' section explains how to carry out the activity in easy stages. The importance of ensuring that all the activities meet the needs of individual children is covered in the last two bullet-pointed ideas, which suggest how to simplify the activity for younger or less able children and how to provide greater challenges for older or more able children.

## Using the photocopiable pages
There are 18 photocopiable pages in this book, of which two are assessment sheets, and sixteen which aim to support or extend the individual activities. None of these photocopiable pages are intended to be used as time-fillers out of context.

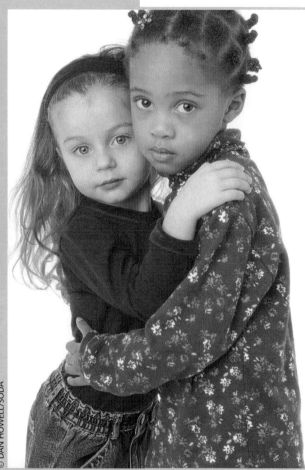

© DAN HOWELL/SODA

## Links with other curriculum areas

The early years Foundation Stage curriculum should not be considered in terms of distinct Areas of Learning. Most activities will provide children with learning opportunities in several Areas of Learning, and making links between these areas is an important part of the planning process. At the end of each activity there is a section called 'Other curriculum areas' which aims to assist practitioners to achieve the same Stepping Stone or Early Learning Goal in a different Area of Learning, thus providing an integrated and sound basis for each child's personal development. These are identified in the shortened form of PSED (Personal, social and emotional development), CLL (Communication, language and literacy), MD (Mathematical development), KUW (Knowledge and understanding of the world), PD (Physical development) and CD (Creative development) to match the six Areas of Learning.

Children's personal, social and emotional development can be considerably enhanced through physical activities. As children experience the enjoyment of exercise, their self-esteem grows, along with their confidence to try greater challenges. This in turn increases well-being and creates a positive approach to a healthy lifestyle. As they master skills in feeding, dressing and personal hygiene, their independence increases, and as they learn, for example, to climb a climbing frame, they experience a satisfying feeling of control over their own bodies. Group activities encourage the social skills of taking turns, sharing, caring and considering others.

The children's communication, language and literacy skills can be extended as they take imaginary journeys, make labels for equipment and talk about experiences.

Through physical activities, mathematical skills will be enhanced as the children are encouraged to count apparatus, measure quantities of sand and sort clothing.

The children's knowledge and understanding of the world can be increased as they explore their surroundings, handle a wide range of natural and made materials, and discover why and how things work.

Creative skills can be developed as the children handle a variety of materials to create their own pictures and models, as well as listen to music while painting.

## Links with home

Each activity provides a 'Home links' section. This encourages parents and carers to be involved in the activity and extend it at home. This section also serves to develop a greater partnership between your setting and the children's homes.

# Planning

### Foundation Stage planning

Good planning for the Foundation Stage is essential in order to ensure that the children are introduced to exciting, challenging and stimulating learning opportunities during their early years. This will form a strong foundation for the children's future education and development. All those involved in creating these opportunities, and supporting the children who have access to them, should work together to promote an effective environment in which maximum learning can take place. This involves developing close partnerships with parents and carers to ensure that strong links between home and setting are established.

Effective planning builds upon children's achievements in small manageable steps from the beginning to the end of the Foundation Stage, so that they become confident, enthusiastic learners. This chapter offers guidance in planning for this progression throughout the Foundation Stage in the area of Physical development.

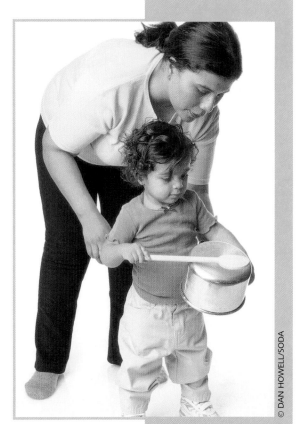

### Planning for a progression of ideas

The *Curriculum Guidance for the Foundation Stage* divides Physical development into five aspects of learning. The activity pages in this book link directly to this document, with each chapter covering one of the aspects of learning.

During the early years, children make rapid strides in their physical development. As they gain control over their movements, so their confidence increases. It is important to plan for this control to develop gradually, so that the children do not attempt strenuous movements before their bodies are physically ready for them. Equally, it is important not to expect too much too soon as the children gain control over fine movement skills such as painting, drawing and writing. The activity 'Painted fences' on page 69, encourages the children to paint fences with large brushes to establish this control gradually.

By the time children reach the age of three, they are becoming increasingly independent in dressing, feeding and personal hygiene. At this stage, they can also be introduced to the importance of a healthy diet and regular exercise. If such experiences are planned as part of the regular routines of your setting, children will come to recognise their importance and develop positive attitudes towards a healthy lifestyle.

Children's physical development is essentially individual, and within any group, rates of development will differ significantly. If the activities that you have planned are too demanding, the children will quickly lose confidence. Conversely, if the activities lack challenge, the children will rapidly lose motivation.

**Physical development**

This book is divided into five chapters, one for each aspect of learning, so that early years practitioners can easily find effective ways of covering all the Early Learning Goals and Stepping Stones within each aspect. This will enable you to decide upon appropriate experiences relevant to the stage of development of individuals rather than chronological age. Each activity includes ideas to support those who are not yet fully confident, or to extend those who require extra challenges.

### Planning for equal opportunities

It is important that all children attending a group setting should feel welcome and know that their contributions are valued. They will have different experiences and interests, and will approach activities with

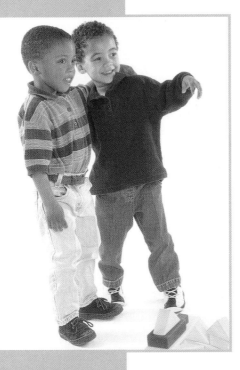

varying skills and knowledge. All the children should have opportunities to benefit from physical activities. Some will approach such experiences with enthusiasm and confidence, while others may be hesitant and worried about getting hurt, preferring the security of familiar experiences. Practitioners need to be aware of this diversity when planning learning activities and experiences. This is particularly important when planning physical activities where challenge, risk and body movements are involved.

It is essential to be aware of requirements on equal opportunities regarding race, gender and disability. These are covered in *The Sex Discrimination Act 1975*, *The Race Relations Act 1976* and *The Disability Discrimination Act 1995*. Planning should also take into account the revised SEN *Code of Practice*, which specifies requirements for intervention in early years settings. The activities in this book are intended to be accessible to all children, but by their nature many will need to be adapted for those with physical disabilities such as reduced mobility and impaired vision. Children with mild or moderate learning difficulties may need to have activities broken down into manageable tasks so that they can feel a sense of achievement as they master these individually, rather than try to complete the whole activity. This may involve modifying instructions or the actual activity. The *Curriculum Guidance for the Foundation Stage* provides advice on pages 17, 18 and 19 about the requirements of providing equal opportunities for all children and how to support planning for children with special educational needs and disabilities to help them make the best possible progress.

### Long-term planning

Long-term planning should provide the framework that underpins the work of your setting, identifying the learning opportunities to be provided over a period of time. These plans might include the Early Learning Goals towards which all work is aimed, the topics planned to link the Areas of Learning or the aspects of learning, and an indication of special events or activities planned to enhance the children's learning, such as religious festivals and local outings.

It is important that all aspects of learning be included and that there be a good balance between and within the Areas of Learning. There

should also be an opportunity to visit aspects of
learning often, on a regular basis, rather than
just once. The aspects of learning for Physical
development are detailed in the introduction of
this book. They are also listed and numbered for
easy reference on page 20 of the QCA
document *Planning for Learning in the
Foundation Stage.*

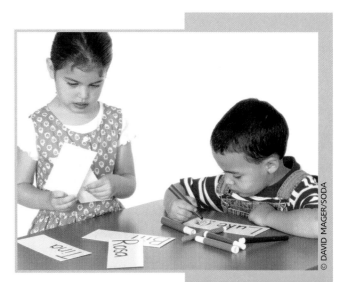

## Medium-term planning

Medium-term planning is a useful indicator of
how the curriculum will be developed over a
shorter period of time, for example, half a term,
and forms a link between the broad overview of
the long-term plan and the more detailed short-
term plans. It should be informed by children's
prior attainment and be sufficiently flexible to meet any changes in the
interests and needs of the children. It is usually based on a topic and
indicates the activities to be used as starting-points to support teaching
and learning intentions within each Area of Learning. It is useful to
identify specific resources needed to arrange and carry out activities at
this stage to assist organisation. Opportunities for assessment may also
be highlighted.

## Short-term planning

Short-term planning demonstrates how the activities that are planned to
meet the learning objectives identified in medium-term planning will be
carried out on a day-to-day or weekly basis. Often such planning includes
the play areas in which activities will take place, whether the activity is
adult-led or child-initiated, and an approximate indication of time. The
Stepping Stones are used at this stage to indicate the different stages of
development as the children progress towards the Early Learning Goals.
Information from discussions, assessments and observations is used to
help to match activities and experiences to the needs of individuals or
groups of children. Any additional requirements to meet those needs are
indicated, for example, reference will sometimes be made as to which
children the staff will focus on or target during specific activities. The
deployment of staff, students and volunteers should be indicated as well
as the grouping of children, if appropriate. Resources to be used can
also be included at this stage in planning rather than within medium-
term plans.

The importance of developing children's communication skills can be
emphasised on short-term planning by including suggestions for
appropriate adult questions and suggested new vocabulary to introduce.

## Organisation

Good organisation is necessary in order to implement plans and activities
effectively, so that the children obtain maximum benefits from the
learning opportunities offered in your setting. This involves defining the
role of the adults involved and considering the layout of the different
play areas.

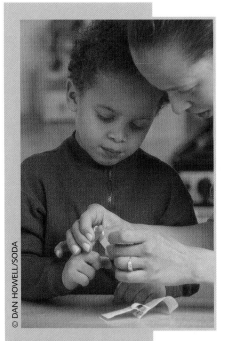

© DAN HOWELL/SODA

### Adults' roles

The main role of the adults within any early years setting is to provide quality support for the children's learning and to ensure that they make appropriate progress in all aspects of their learning and development. It is essential that as much of their time as possible is spent working directly with the children. This involves interacting effectively during play and learning experiences, for example, giving praise, explaining things clearly, asking challenging questions and extending the children's ideas.

The number of staff will vary from setting to setting. A childminder may work alone, while a manager in a day nursery will be responsible for the selection and recruitment of a number of staff. In all cases, sharing ideas, difficulties and successes is a necessary part of developing a quality learning environment. If there are insufficient staff members, a support group could be set up for such a purpose. It is necessary for all staff to be aware of their roles, so that they can make a clear contribution to the children's security, welfare, learning and development. Individual strengths, interests and skills should be utilised to extend opportunities and introduce new experiences.

### Key workers

Some settings appoint key workers to be responsible for the welfare of a small group of children. These staff members are familiar faces for parents and carers to turn to, to discuss any concerns or successes that their children might have. In addition, key workers often have responsibility for maintaining a child's assessment details and share these regularly on a one-to-one basis with the parents or carers.

### Staff meetings

Regular staff meetings are an important part of organisation and allow staff to voice any concerns that they may have. These meetings are also a time to decide upon any action over unexpected problems that might arise, whether organisational, domestic or child-related.

Larger nurseries may include regular times in the day when the children work or enjoy snacks and meals with their key workers in small groups. This encourages a sense of belonging. Others might organise the children into groups with particular names, such as 'robins' and 'sparrows', and these groups may work with different staff members rather than key workers.

### Regular routines

Underpinning all well-organised early years settings is a clear structure and daily routine. Children feel relaxed and secure when they know 'what is coming next'. They will enter the setting eagerly, confident about how the session will start and what is expected of them. As the day progresses, they will be comfortable about routines such as snacks and mealtimes, and be able to find any resources that they need for their chosen activities. They will join in with clearing up and take part in farewell routines. Staff should work as a team to create these regular routines and support any children who seem anxious, particularly new children. The importance of daily routines associated with a healthy lifestyle are emphasised in Chapter 3 of this book.

## Setting up a suitable play environment

Staff will be able to give more time to working directly with the children if the environment is planned effectively. All staff should be involved in organising a safe, well-structured environment that allows the children freedom to explore, investigate and follow their interests. Familiarity with the layout of your room is encouraged in the activity 'Clever messengers' on page 34, in which the children should be able to work independently. The activity 'I can manage!' on page 78 encourages the children to develop familiarity with storage and organisation of resources and the activity 'Tidy-up time!' on page 38 involves the children in learning to be responsible for their own environment.

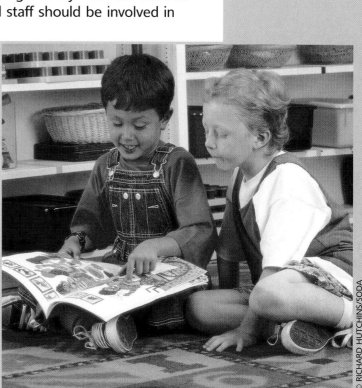

Resources should be made available for a suitable amount of time so that the children can return to them to reinforce their ideas and try out new ones.

When setting up a suitable play environment for physical development, it is essential to consider the safety aspects involved in the free exploration mentioned above – for example, constant supervision is required on climbing apparatus. The activity 'Follow the rules' on page 37 involves the children in creating their own set of rules for using large apparatus safely. The children also need to be shown how to handle tools correctly, such as scissors. The activity 'Working with wood' on page 74 explores safe handling of woodwork tools.

### Outdoor areas

Some activities require a large space in which the children can move freely and gain control over their body movements. This may not always be possible indoors, so planning appropriate use of the outdoor environment for physical activities is as important as organising indoor play areas. Organise the area into different sections so that, for example, those riding bicycles will not be near to those playing with balls.

Ideally there should be:
■ an empty space for role-play related to the current theme or the children's own ideas (for example, the activity 'Trains, boats and places' on page 19 involves setting up a Noah's Ark role-play activity)
■ an area to ride wheeled vehicles (for example, the activity 'Drive carefully!' on page 31 encourages the children to ride along chalk pathways)
■ a defined space to play with small apparatus (for example, the activity 'Knock them flat!' on page 36 introduces games using home-made skittles)

# Planning

■ a space set out for large apparatus with appropriate mats provided if there is not a safety surface (for example, the activity 'Baby crows' on page 23 involves the children jumping off benches on to safety mats)
■ a small area with opportunities to develop manipulative skills, for example, a painting easel in fine weather
■ a clear space for planned activities (for example, the activity 'Trains, planes and boats' on page 19 encourages the children to move freely as different vehicles).

Settings without an outdoor area need to allocate a clear indoor space for more vigorous physical activities for at least part of every session. It may not be possible to define separate areas indoors because of lack of space, so opportunities for physical play should be planned carefully each week to allow for different opportunities.

## Play areas

Sand and water can be enjoyed both indoors and outdoors, but ensure that outdoor sand is covered when it is not in use, so that animals cannot reach it. Introduce a range of equipment of different shapes and sizes, for example, graded funnels and measuring scoops, to develop small movement skills such as pouring, grasping, lifting and turning.

The activity 'Forest camp' on page 39 invites the children to role-play and involves a range of large and small movements as they create a forest camp.

Small-world play is encouraged in the activity 'Down on the farm' on page 72, where the children can develop fine finger and hand movements as they create a farm layout.

The activity 'Wriggling snakes' on page 42 gives the children the opportunity to carry out craft activities, developing their manipulative skills as they thread pasta to create wriggling snakes.

Natural discovery can help the children to develop both their small and large body movements as they plant beans and imitate their growth by moving their own bodies in the fun activity 'Full of beans!' on page 21.

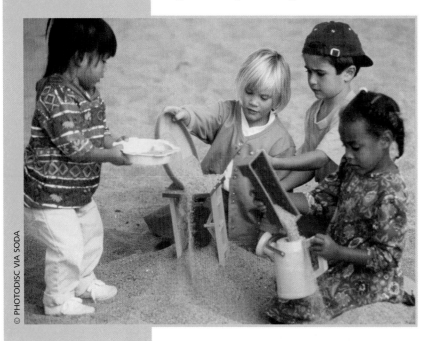

The activity 'Parking places' on page 71 offers opportunities to develop manipulative skills as the children construct garages for their cars.

Malleable materials are used in the activity 'Fun with dough' on page 75, which invites the children to prepare their own play dough using a range of small movement skills.

Finally, the ICT area is at the centre of the musical activity 'Mood music' on page 22, where a tape recorder or CD player can be used to provide music for the children to express free movement.

**Physical development**

# Assessment

### The importance of assessment

Assessment is an essential part of the role of early years practitioners during the Foundation Stage. It enables them to identify when individuals or groups of children have achieved the knowledge, skills and attitudes that are needed to move on to the next steps in their learning.

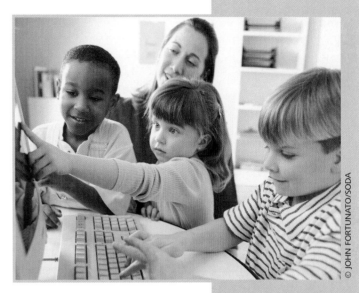

Early years practitioners begin to assess children informally from when they first enter a setting, as they interact with them in their work and play. They are able to observe their day-to-day progress, share their experiences and find out about their interests. As time passes, they begin to understand the children's individual ways of learning, discover their preferences, celebrate their achievements and help them to overcome their difficulties. However, in order to ensure that all aspects of a child's development are monitored carefully, this informal assessment needs to work alongside a formal system.

Assessing children's attainment and progress is an integral part of the planning cycle, helping staff to build successfully upon what a child already knows and is interested in, and identifying any gaps in their knowledge. Staff can then confidently steer a child towards new learning and ensure that the activities and experiences that they plan and organise become successful learning opportunities. Once plans are put into practice, staff can observe and record the children's progress as they take part in the activities and experiences provided. This will enable them to adjust future plans, for example, to give the children additional support or provide them with greater challenges.

It is important to make an initial assessment of a child's stage of development on entry to your setting, or perhaps during a home visit, as a basis for planning appropriate activities for that child, and to follow this up with a more formal initial assessment once the child has settled in. Regular formative assessments can then be made to give a picture of a child's progress over a longer term. Assessment opportunities can be identified initially on medium-term plans, ensuring that there is a good balance across the six Areas of Learning. Short-term plans can then be used to indicate when, where and how assessment will take place, together with the names of staff and children involved.

A summative assessment will provide evidence of a child's stage of development on leaving the setting.

### Involving parents and carers

Parents and carers should be involved with assessment from when their child first enters your setting. For example, when considering physical

**Physical development**

development, their contributions will be more effective if they are given information to increase their understanding of the Early Learning Goals for Physical development, and details of significant developmental milestones. Assessment should not only be a partnership between staff and parents and carers, but should also include the children and any relevant outside agencies, such as health professionals. This partnership is particularly important when a child has a special educational need and an individual educational plan (IEP) needs to be created.

## Observation

Observation is an essential part of the overall planning and assessment system. When considering physical development, it is a means of discovering what a child is physically capable of doing at any given time, rather than making assumptions based on what that child is expected to be doing. Observing closely and listening intently, as children work and play, provides the practitioner with more valuable evidence than analysing the end product of their actions. Appropriate documentation should be produced, which will serve to build up a picture of a child's progress over time. There are many ways of conducting observations and these are often a personal preference of a setting. However, it is important that all members of staff be involved.

### Planning an observation

When planning an observation, adults should ensure that they have time to focus on an individual or group of children, and to share the results of their observations with their colleagues. Observers should not be intrusive but stand back, listen attentively and watch, without distracting the child or group of children. If necessary, they should ask the children appropriate questions or discuss problems that they might encounter in order to get a fuller picture of a child's understanding of a situation. Observations should always be written down, for example, in a diary or on an observation sheet, and a system for jotting down spontaneous observations to write up later, such as Post-it notes, would be useful. It is important to record the actual language that the children use.

There are many appropriate things to observe in a busy setting that will provide evidence of the children's progress, and all staff should be involved in the process. Identify when observations will be made on planning and ensure that they are manageable and part of the daily routine.

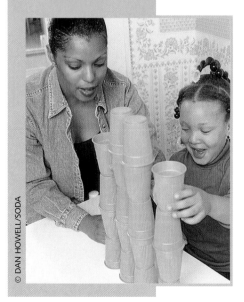

© DAN HOWELL/SODA

### Observing the children

When carrying out an observation, consider the following:
■ individual children, working alone, in pairs, small friendship groups or with an adult
■ the children's response to an activity
■ indoor and outdoor play areas within your setting to evaluate efficiency of organisation and resourcing
■ a particular aspect of a child's development in order to build up an overall picture over time
■ the children's social interactions, language development or physical skills.

## Observation methods

Individual tracking is a useful method of following a child's movements. Note the frequency of visits to the different play areas and any areas that the child chooses to avoid. Use the information to build up a picture of a child's individuality and stage of development.

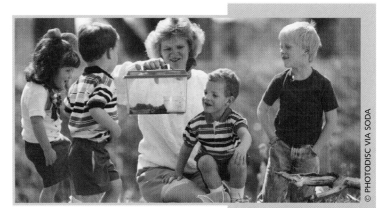

Individual observations are a more detailed way of observing a child's response to an activity and the language used. It is an effective means of identifying what a child can actually do in order to plan for future progression. Extra observations can be planned if there are specific concerns about an aspect of a child's development.

Observing small group activities is a good way to identify any children who need extra support, or any that are ready for further challenges.

## Methods of record keeping

Records celebrate and demonstrate what a child can do at a given time. This enables staff to plan appropriate activities to ensure that the child moves with confidence to the next stage in their development. Keeping records will identify significant skills or difficulties so that staff, parents and carers and other professionals can work together to meet the needs of those children who require additional challenge or support. Record keeping should be manageable and easily understood, as well as being shared readily with a child's parents or carers. There is no ideal system for record keeping, but it is important that staff, parents and carers should feel comfortable with the personal system that they develop. Children should be consulted, if appropriate, perhaps in deciding on favourite pieces of work to include in their portfolios.

## Recording physical development

The following is a guide to successful record keeping:

■ include personal records giving essential details related to a child, such as medical and dietary needs

■ ask parents or carers to fill in an initial record of achievement before a child enters your setting

■ use target sheets of expected physical achievements, with a space to tick or highlight once a target is achieved; however this method can be misleading if used in isolation as adults may make inaccurate assumptions

■ carry out regular recordings of observation of the children's activities, behaviour and use of language

■ complete summative assessment sheets, often supplied by local authorities, prior to the child's entry to school

■ date samples of work and photographs of activities indicating a child's progress over a period of time

■ tape-record and video the children's conversations as these are especially useful for monitoring language and social development

■ include key worker or individual staff records

■ send written reports to parents and carers.

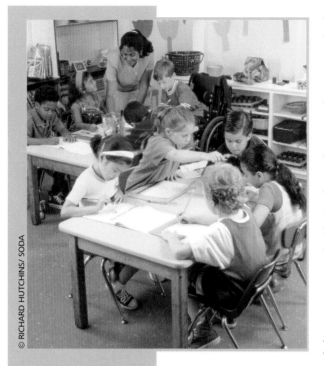

© RICHARD HUTCHINS/ SODA

## Assessing physical development

Assessment, using a combination of the above methods, can provide practitioners with an overall picture of a child's physical development during the Foundation Stage. It is also a means of checking that the Stepping Stones and Early Learning Goals have been covered comprehensively. If a child is experiencing difficulty, for example, with handling tools such as scissors, additional activities can be planned to enable the child to develop this skill through varied experiences. Assessment will also draw attention to any children who may have special educational needs, so that support and advice can be obtained from appropriate professionals.

## Foundation Stage Profile

In January 2003, the Qualifications and Curriculum Authority introduced a new assessment document for early years practitioners working within the Foundation Stage. The *Foundation Stage Profile* provides a 12-page document to be completed for each child throughout the Foundation Stage. Within it the curriculum is broken down to provide assessment for all six Areas of Learning. For the area of Physical development, there are nine 'targets'.

Practitioners will be expected to use their usual techniques of observation and occasional note taking to gather evidence of the children's skills and abilities. They will be required to make a note of the date when a child fulfils a target and make comments.

## Using this book for assessment

The photocopiable assessment sheets on pages 79 and 80 are designed to provide a means of recording the children's physical progress throughout the Foundation Stage. The sheets provide details of the Early Learning Goals that the children need to achieve by the end of this stage. Space has been provided on each sheet for you to make notes and observations about individual children's progress.

The following example demonstrates how the assessment sheets can be used to indicate a child's progress. The activity 'Noah's Ark' on page 30 invites the children to pretend to be animals going into Noah's Ark. The learning objective is to move like animals, thus 'I can imitate the movements of other living creatures'. This leads to the Stepping Stone 'Move in a range of ways, such as slithering, shuffling, rolling, crawling, walking, running, jumping, skipping, sliding and hopping', which in turn leads to the Early Learning Goal 'Move with confidence, imagination and in safety'. The learning objective is unique to the activity, but there may be other activities covering the same Stepping Stone, and several visiting the Early Learning Goal.

By using this system, a child is able to revisit the Early Learning Goals in different stimulating and exciting ways regularly throughout the Foundation Stage.

This chapter provides ideas to encourage the children to move with confidence and imagination as well as in safety, to develop control over and co-ordination of movements, and to travel around, under, over and through balancing and climbing equipment.

# Trains, boats and planes

## What to do

■ Explore the display with the children and encourage them to pick up the resources freely and look at the pictures. Talk about the different modes of transport.

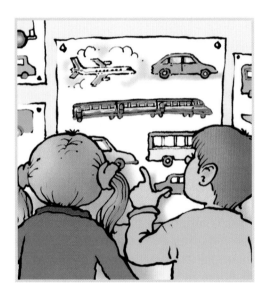

■ Sit on the floor in an open space. Introduce the word 'transport' and invite the children to talk about their experiences of travelling by road, sea and air.

■ Decide on a familiar form of travel and suggest that the children move around the open space pretending to be that mode of transport. Would their passengers have a smooth or bumpy ride? Would they be in the air, on the ground or on the sea?

■ Explore different examples of transport so that the children can move in straight lines, around corners, and up and down.

■ Ensure that all the children move safely by emphasising the need to look out for others while they are moving, to avoid collisions.

■ Give younger children lots of praise for individual movement variations to encourage them to express their imagination with confidence.

■ With older children, discuss safety procedures associated with travel, such as fastening seat belts and stopping at warning lights. Develop role-play to combine these situations with appropriate movement activities.

## More ideas

■ Use tables draped with fabric to create tunnels for an underground tube or a Channel Tunnel train to crawl through.

■ Encourage the children's imaginary movements by exploring unusual travel such as riding on camels or being pulled by a team of huskies.

## Other curriculum areas

PSED  Create a role-play train and invite passengers to take turns to come aboard for an imaginary journey.

CLL  Sing 'transport' rhymes with actions, such as 'The Wheels on the Bus' and 'Aeroplanes, Aeroplanes, All in a Row' both from *This Little Puffin...* compiled by Elizabeth Matterson (Puffin Books) .

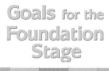

**Goals** for the **Foundation Stage**

**Stepping Stone**
Move spontaneously within available space.

**Early Learning Goal**
Move with confidence, imagination and in safety.

**Group size**
Up to eight children.

**What you need**
Table; pictures and books showing different modes of transport; small-world vehicles; large open space.

**Preparation**
Arrange the books and small-world vehicles on a table, with the pictures behind.

**Home links**
Invite parents and carers to bring in photographs of their children travelling on different modes of transport. Suggest that parents and carers pretend to go on imaginary journeys with their children.

# Out in all weathers

**Early Learning Goal**
Move with confidence, imagination and in safety.

**Group size**
Up to eight children.

**What you need**
Selection of percussion instruments; sheets of thick card; cardboard tubes; chiffon scarves; tape recorder or CD player; tapes or CDs of music such as the 'Thunderstorm' movement from Beethoven's *Pastoral Symphony*.

**Preparation**
Ask for permisson from parents and carers to take the children for walks in different weathers.

**Home links**
Give each child a copy of the photocopiable sheet 'Weather rhymes' on page 81 to share with their parents and carers at home.

## What to do
■ Take the children for walks in different weathers. Draw their attention to what they can see, hear and feel.
■ Back at your setting, make comparisons between walking in wind, rain and sun. What do rain and wind sound like? How do they feel? Is it harder to walk in wind or rain?
■ Invite each child to choose an instrument to play and talk about the sounds that they make.
■ Play the instruments while the children listen. Do any have a simple repetitive beat that

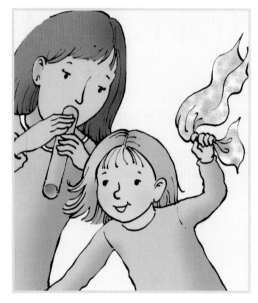

reminds them of raindrops? Try to re-create the sound of the wind, for example, by rattling a sheet of card or blowing down a cardboard tube.
■ Encourage the children to move freely to contrasting sounds such as a shaking tambourine and a clacking castanet.
■ Invite some children to invent 'wind' sounds from objects or instruments, while others pretend to be the wind by running around using twisting and turning movements. Emphasise the effect by giving them chiffon scarves to hold while they are moving around.
■ Ask some children to re-create raindrop movements while others make rhythmic sounds for them to move to.
■ Encourage younger children to move like raindrops when they hear the beat of an instrument, and stand still when there is no sound.
■ Introduce older children to music related to the weather such as the 'Thunderstorm' movement from Beethoven's *Pastoral Symphony*, and invite them to move freely to the music.

## More ideas
■ Use the children's experiences of walking in the rain as a starting-point to dramatise the story of *Noah's Ark* (*Usborne Bible Tales*, Usborne Publishing).
■ Act out rhymes associated with weather, such as 'Doctor Foster Went to Gloucester' (Traditional).

### Other curriculum areas
CD — Beat an instrument and encourage the children to paint 'rainy' pictures as they listen.
CLL — Read *The Wind Blew* by Pat Hutchins (Red Fox) and let the children move like the objects and characters in the story.

**Physical development**

# Full of beans!

## What to do

■ Talk with the children about how the seeds germinated using movement words such as 'pushed', 'poked' and 'popped'. Discuss how the emerging seedlings stretch up through the compost towards the light and how the leaves gradually unroll from the stalk.

■ Suggest that the children pretend to be the bean seeds tightly curled up in the compost. Discuss the sequence of movement as the seed germinates and grows into a strong bean plant.

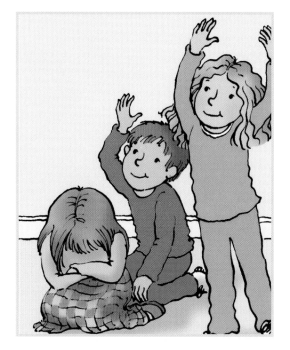

■ Use appropriate words to 'tell the story' of the bean. Encourage the children to use appropriate movements to act out the story as you tell it. Pause to praise the children's individual movements and to suggest new movements such as waving and making tall or wide shapes.

■ Work alongside younger children. If they are anxious, emphasise that you are happy for them to sit and watch until they feel ready to take part.

■ Invite older children to re-enact the story of 'Jack and the Beanstalk' (Traditional) with emphasis on the growth of the beanstalk.

## More ideas

■ Carry out other movements involving sequence, for example, pretending to get dressed in the morning.

■ Set up an obstacle course and encourage the children to move across it in different ways.

## Other curriculum areas

CLL Act out the rhyme 'I Had a Little Cherry Stone' from *This Little Puffin...* compiled by Elizabeth Matterson (Puffin Books) using finger movements, then body movements.

KUW Experiment with the growth of a variety of seeds and plants, and demonstrate observations of any differences through body movements.

### Home links
Explain the learning objective of the activity to parents and carers. Suggest how they might make up appropriate actions and sequences of movement with their children as they sing rhymes and songs together at home.

Physical development

# Mood music

**Early Learning Goal**
Move with confidence, imagination and in safety.

**Group size**
Up to eight children.

**What you need**
CD player or tape recorder; selection of CDs or tapes of music to evoke moods such as the 'Thunderstorm' movement from Beethoven's *Pastoral Symphony* (angry), *The Flight of the Bumble Bee* by Rimsky-Korsakov (exciting) and 'Fossils' (happy) and 'The Swan' (sad) from *Carnival of the Animals* by Saint-Saëns.

**Preparation**
Choose pieces of music to play to represent contrasting moods beforehand and make a note of the CD tracks or position on the tapes.

## What to do
■ Talk to the children about what makes them feel angry, excited, happy and sad.
■ Explain to the children that you are going to listen to some music together and suggest that they make themselves comfortable in a space so that they can listen without interruption. Some children might like to lie down while others will prefer to sit up.

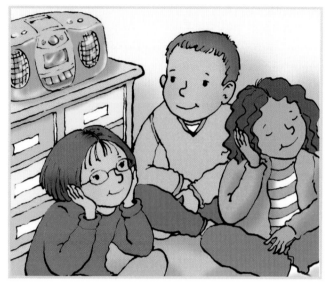

■ Start by playing a rousing, exciting piece of music to attract the children's interest. Talk about how the music made them feel. Was it fast or slow, loud or quiet?
■ Listen to each piece of music in turn, ending with slow, dreamy music to make the children feel relaxed.
■ Invite the children to invent dances to show how the different music makes them feel.
■ Modify the selection of music if younger children are overwhelmed by very loud, emotional music.
■ Let older children take turns to make up a 'feelings dance' without music, and see if the others can guess the depicted mood.

## More ideas
■ Supply a selection of musical instruments, streamers, scarves and ribbons for the children to use during their dances.
■ Dramatise traditional stories involving a range of emotions, for example, 'The Three Billy Goats Gruff', 'Goldilocks and the Three Bears' and 'Jack and the Beanstalk' (Traditional).

**Home links**
Suggest to parents and carers that they encourage their children to make up dances at home while listening to different types of music. Emphasise the importance of talking about how the music makes them feel.

## Other curriculum areas
PSED Invite the children to make faces into mirrors to depict different emotions, such as happy, surprised, angry and sad, then make paper-plate collage faces to add to a 'feelings' display.

CD Encourage the children to paint pictures while listening to the music selection prepared for the main activity.

# Baby crows

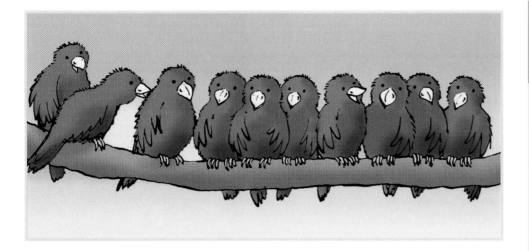

## What to do

■ Read the 'Little learners' number rhyme on the photocopiable sheet to the children and talk to them about how adult birds look after their young and teach them to fly.

■ Show the children the bench and ask them to imagine that this is a branch of a tree. Invite the children to be the baby crows sitting along the branch.

■ Before you read the rhyme, demonstrate to the children how to jump off the bench on to the safety mat, landing on two feet and bending at the knees. Then pretend to fly around the open space surrounding the bench and sit down away from the safety mat.

■ As you read each verse, ask one of the 'baby crows' to jump from the bench to the safety mat before flying around the open space, then sit beside the other children on the floor.

■ If younger children are apprehensive about jumping by themselves, hold a hand to steady them until they feel confident.

■ Older children will enjoy the challenge of walking along the bench and jumping off the end instead of sitting in a row.

## More ideas

■ Create opportunities for the children to jump off apparatus on to safety mats as part of an obstacle course.

■ Introduce jumping into role-play, for example, jumping off a 'pirate ship' into the 'deep, blue sea'.

### Other curriculum areas

MD  Make number cards to attach to the baby crows in the rhyme and count how many birds are left on the branch after each verse.

PSED  Discuss the importance of taking turns to jump off the bench to avoid collisions. Then introduce further opportunities to take turns by playing group games.

### Stepping Stone
Jump off an object and land appropriately.

### Early Learning Goal
Move with confidence, imagination and in safety.

■

### Group size
Five children.

■

### What you need
The photocopiable sheet 'Little learners' on page 82 ; low bench; safety mat.

■

### Preparation
Arrange the bench alongside a safety mat.

### Home links
Encourage parents and carers to develop their children's movement skills by finding safe opportunities for them to jump from objects on to safe surfaces, for example, soft-play apparatus. Explain the importance of landing on two feet and bending at the knees.

# All wrapped up

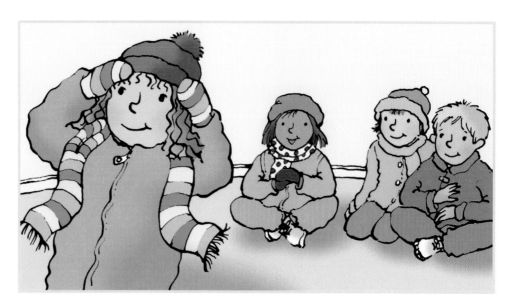

## What to do

■ Ask the children to put on their outdoor coats and sit on the floor in a row at one end of a large space.

■ Put a hat, scarf and pair of mittens for each child in a large pile at the other end of the floor space.

■ Explain to the children that when they hear a given signal, for example, a clap of your hands, the first child should run to the other end of the floor space and choose a hat, scarf and pair of mittens to put on before returning to the back of the row and sitting down again. The next child should repeat these actions, and play continues until all the children have had a turn and are dressed in outdoor clothing.

■ If the children manage this easily, introduce a large sand-timer and try to complete the activity before the sand runs out. Reduce the number of children if those who are waiting become restless.

■ Run about outdoors for a few minutes, if possible, before returning indoors to take off the clothing.

■ Let younger children sit in a circle with the clothes in the centre and take turns to choose a hat and put it on until all are wearing hats. Repeat with the scarves and then the mittens.

■ Challenge older children to play the game in two teams, and include gloves instead of mittens.

## Other curriculum areas

**MD** Let the children play a game by putting clothes on in the correct sequence.

**PSED** Allocate an older child to help a younger child to dress for outdoor play.

## More ideas

■ Play a similar game involving changing from indoor shoes to wellington boots.

■ Introduce into the role-play area a variety of dressing-up clothes and dolls' clothes that have different types of fastenings.

**Physical development**

# Beanbag balance

## What to do

■ Begin by asking the children to find a space of their own and to sit on the floor. Which parts of their bodies can they touch from this position? Can they touch their toes, their backs, under their knees?

■ Encourage the children to stand up with their hands by their sides and then to stretch their arms above their heads, out to the side and back down again.

■ How long can the children stand on one leg by counting seconds? Is the time the same on the other leg?

■ Invite the children to choose a beanbag from the storage container and find a space again.

■ Talk to the children about the meaning of the word 'balance' and tell them that they are going to try balancing the beanbags on different parts of their bodies. Can they walk about with a beanbag on their head?

■ Ask younger children to lie down and try balancing the beanbag on a hand while lifting up their arm.

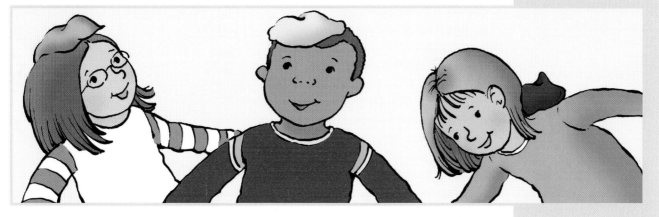

■ Let older children explore their own balancing ideas with the beanbags and take turns to show them to the rest of the group.

## More ideas

■ Use other small apparatus such as quoits or light plastic balls to explore balance.

■ Have egg-and-spoon races using golf balls instead of eggs.

### Other curriculum ideas

**KUW** Encourage the children to name the different parts of their bodies as they try to touch them from a sitting position or balance their beanbags on them.

**MD** Show the children how to use a ball of string to measure how far they can walk with a beanbag on their heads.

# Let's go home!

**Early Learning Goal**
Move with control and co-ordination.

**Group size**
Four children.

**What you need**
The photocopiable sheet 'Find the way home' on page 83; card; laminator; glue; dice; small-world figures; selection of board games that use dice.

**Preparation**
If possible, make an enlarged copy of the photocopiable sheet, glue it on to a piece of card and laminate it for protection. Make a table display of the selection of games.

**Home links**
Ask parents and carers to loan board games for the display and encourage them to play dice games at home with their children.

## What to do

■ Look at the selection of games and talk about the children's favourites. Why do they like these games? Can they explain how to play them? What movements are involved?

■ Show the children the gameboard. Explain that the object of the game is to move from the school building at one end of the road to the house at the other. Ask the children to suggest any other resources that you might need in order to play the game, and gather these together.

■ Put a small-world figure next to the school building on the gameboard and ask the children to take turns to throw the dice and move the figure the corresponding number of spaces along the path to the house at the other end.

■ Younger children will find playing the game easier and more exciting if they sit on the floor and throw a large sponge dice instead of a normal dice.

■ Let older children enjoy the challenge of having a figure each and seeing which is first to arrive 'home'.

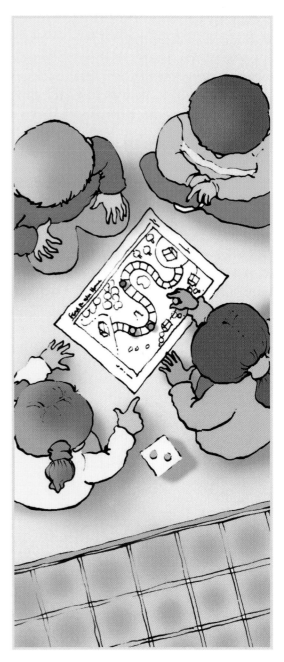

## More ideas

■ Make your own dice of different sizes using wooden blocks, large foam cubes and tiny plastic cubes. Add stickers to depict the numbers.

■ Play games to develop the children's manipulative skills, such as trying to thread as many beads as possible on to a lace before a sand-timer runs out.

### Other curriculum areas

MD ■ Invite the children to design their own gameboards and make dice.

KUW ■ Create board games related to a topic, such as animals in a forest finding their way home.

# Which way will you go?

## What to do
- Ask the children to sit on the floor while you explain any safety rules for using the apparatus, then allow time for free exploration.
- Invite the children to sit down again and talk about what they have been doing. Ask appropriate questions to introduce different

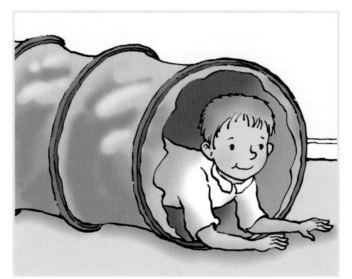

ways of moving, for example, 'Did anyone crawl forwards through the tunnel?' and 'Did anyone climb over the bench?'.
- Suggest that the children choose a piece of apparatus, then move among them, acknowledging and praising them for completing appropriate movements, for example, 'You managed to climb up these steps easily' and 'I noticed you slithering under the bench'.
- Simplify tasks for younger children and praise them for their attempts, however easy they may seem.
- Challenge older children to move in different ways, asking them, for example, 'Have you tried crawling backwards through the tunnel?' and 'Can you walk sideways along the bench?'.

## More ideas
- Set up apparatus to depict an imaginary journey, for example, inviting the children to cross a bridge made from a bench, and to climb up and down a steep mountain represented by a slide.
- Create an imaginary role-play jungle using a range of apparatus.

## Other curriculum areas
**MD** Use positional language while the children are playing with construction equipment by asking them to put pieces in specific places, for example, 'on top of the tower' and 'inside the box'.

**PSED** Play games involving taking turns to cross the apparatus.

### Home links
Explain to parents and carers the importance of developing different movement skills, and suggest that they encourage their children to move in different ways on large apparatus in their gardens at home or when visiting a park.

### Stepping Stone
Manage body to create intended movements.

### Early Learning Goal
Travel around, under, over and through balancing and climbing equipment.

### Group size
Up to six children.

### What you need
Selection of large apparatus such as a slide, bench, tunnel and wooden climbing steps; safety mats.

### Preparation
Arrange the apparatus around the room with a safe distance between each piece of equipment. Ensure that safety mats are in appropriate positions. Consider the variety of movements needed to negotiate the apparatus. Make sure that there are opportunities to travel around, under, over and through the items. Add additional apparatus if necessary, so that all these movements are possible.

# Ups and downs

## Stepping Stone
Mount stairs, steps or climbing equipment using alternate feet.

### Early Learning Goal
Travel around, under, over and through balancing and climbing equipment.

### Group size
Four children.

### What you need
Wooden or plastic climbing apparatus in the form of steps; safety mat.

### What to do
■ Discuss the importance of climbing steps carefully and ask the children if they think that they could climb your flight of steps and jump off safely. Explain the importance of landing on two feet when jumping down.

■ Ask the children to sit near to the steps and say the following rhyme:

We can climb right up the steps, one, two and three,
Then we jump back down again, one, two and three!

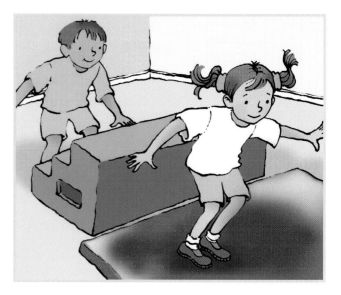

■ Invite a child to climb up and say the rhyme at the same time, substituting 'we' for the child's name. Take turns until all the children have had fun climbing up the steps and jumping on to the safety mat.

■ If you do not have access to 'step' climbing apparatus, look for safe options to practise climbing stairs, but omit the jumping aspect.

■ Hold younger children's hands or stand near by to give them added confidence.

■ Develop more challenging opportunities for older children, perhaps by joining two sets of steps together so that they can climb up and down. Alter the second line of the rhyme to 'Then we climb back down again, one, two and three!'.

### More ideas
■ Act out the rhyme 'Humpty Dumpty' (Traditional) using climbing steps to represent the wall and large floor cushions on top of a safety mat to break Humpty's fall.

■ Arrange two sets of climbing steps back to back to form a hill. Dramatise the rhyme 'The Grand Old Duke of York' (Traditional), taking turns to climb up the hill and come back down again.

### Home links
Encourage parents and carers to make climbing stairs at home a fun activity for the children, for example, by counting or saying a rhyme.

### Other curriculum areas
**CLL** Extend the children's vocabulary by discussing steps and flights of stairs. Talk about steps into cellars, attics and gardens, and make comparisons between bungalows and houses. Discuss their experiences of very long flights of stairs, for example, into an aeroplane.

**KUW** Make steps using construction equipment or recyclable materials.

# Over the hill

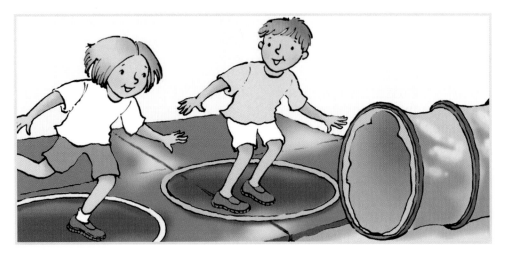

## What to do

■ Share the story 'What a journey!' on the photocopiable sheet with the children and suggest that you act it out together. Explain that one floor cushion is the old house, the other cushion is the new house, and the things in between will need to be crossed during the journey.

■ Read the first part of the story, then suggest that the children take turns to play the part of Isla and the cat, and make the journey to the new home. As you read, pause to introduce appropriate movements if necessary, for example, as the cat negotiates the wide river, deep tunnel and tall hill.

■ Ensure that the obstacles created for younger children are sufficient to challenge them while still being appropriate to their ability.

■ Invite older children to choose the apparatus to use to represent the various challenges met by the characters.

## More ideas

■ Play 'Stations', with 'hopping', 'jumping' and 'sitting' stations. When the children arrive at the stations, they should move in the way indicated by the station name.

■ Play 'Musical statues'. Instruct the children to move around in different ways when the music plays, and to stand or sit still when the music stops.

## Other curriculum areas

CLL Dramatise other favourite stories involving journeys, such as *We're Going on a Bear Hunt* by Michael Rosen (Walker Books) in a similar way.

CD Take turns to pretend to move like an animal and see if the other children can guess which one it is.

### Home links
Give each child a copy of the photocopiable sheet to take home and suggest to parents and carers that they act out the story with their children.

### Stepping Stone
Sit up, stand up and balance on various parts of the body.

### Early Learning Goal
Move with control and co-ordination.

### Group size
Six children.

### What you need
The photocopiable sheet 'What a journey!' on page 84; safety mats (river); plastic tunnel; two sets of climbing steps (hill); hoops (stepping-stones); soft-play shapes (trees and rocks); two large floor cushions.

### Preparation
Arrange the apparatus to depict the obstacles negotiated by Isla in the story 'What a journey!' by putting a floor cushion at each end to represent the old home and the new home. If you do not have soft-play shapes, substitute cushions or similar objects. Make sure that there are opportunities to sit up, stand and balance on various parts of the body when arranging the apparatus.

# Noah's Ark

## What to do

■ Read the story of *Noah's Ark* and ask the children to tell you which is their favourite animal and why.

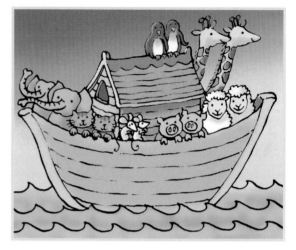

■ Suggest that you make an Ark from construction or soft-play equipment. Arrange the equipment to form the walls of the Ark, large enough for all the children to sit in. Decide how the animals will get into the Ark, perhaps by creating steps or a ramp from the equipment available. Place the dolls inside to appear as Noah and his family, and surround the ark with blue fabric to represent the water.

■ Invite each child to choose which animal they would like to be and ask them to sit around the edge of the 'water' until it is their turn to climb into the Ark.

■ Tell the story in your own words so that you can include the animals chosen by the children. As you mention each animal, use appropriate vocabulary to describe the movement of that animal, based on those indicated within the Stepping Stone, for example, 'the snake slithered', 'the hippopotamus shuffled', 'the frog hopped' and so on.

■ Support younger children by moving with them if necessary. Emphasise that they can sit and watch, either from inside or outside the Ark, until they feel ready to take part.

■ Invite older children to take turns to tell the story while the others act it out.

## More ideas

■ Create a role-play zoo and encourage the children to consider how the different animals will move.

■ Play the music of movements from *Carnival of the Animals* by Saint-Saëns and encourage the children to move freely.

## Other curriculum areas

**CLL** Take photographs of the children moving like animals and add them to a display. Include suitable word labels to describe the children's movements.

**CD** Sing 'Old MacDonald Had a Farm' (Traditional) and invite the children to make appropriate sounds and movements as they represent the different animals.

**Physical development**

While taking part in the activities presented in this chapter, the children will begin to develop an awareness of their personal space and of the space of those around them, within both open and confined spaces.

# Drive carefully!

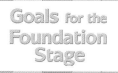

## What to do

▇ Take the children outdoors and invite them to explore the pathways by walking along them in the same direction and using wheelchairs and mobility aids, if appropriate. What happens if some of the children walk the other way? Do they have to move in a different way to pass one another?

▇ Invite the children to try to move in different ways, such as hopping, jumping or running along the paths.

▇ Back indoors, find a clear, carpeted space and suggest that the children each pretend to be a vehicle of their choice, moving freely around the space.

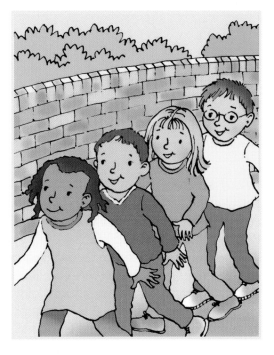

▇ Talk about the surfaces that vehicles travel upon and suggest that the children use the resources that you have available to make a short train track or road, for example, by taping parallel lengths of string securely to the carpet to form a road, or creating a train track from two rows of balance beams. Avoid the possibility of tripping by asking the children to move between bricks, beams and string rather than over them.

▇ Make simple tracks with a 'Start' and a 'Finish' point for younger children to avoid collisions on route.

▇ Encourage older children to show awareness of the movements of others by creating a two-way track.

## Other curriculum areas

CLL Go on an imaginary journey, perhaps for a picnic or on holiday.

KUW Invite a crossing patrol officer to visit your setting to extend safety awareness through role-play using the tracks created.

## More ideas

▇ Make available opportunities for the children to stop and start, such as petrol stations and train stations, and introduce junctions, road signs or signals to follow.

▇ Create a maze and invite the children to find a route across it.

**Stepping Stone**
Negotiate an appropriate pathway when walking, running or using a wheelchair or other mobility aids, both indoors and outdoors.

**Early Learning Goal**
Show awareness of space, of themselves and of others.

▇

**Group size**
Six children.

▇

**What you need**
Outdoor area; thick pieces of chalk; resources to create indoor pathways, such as thick string, masking tape, large plastic bricks and balance beams.

▇

**Preparation**
Using thick chalk, create straight and curved pathways on a hard surface outdoors, wide enough to accommodate wheelchairs or mobility aids, if appropriate. Make use of any existing painted markings.

**Home links**
Explain the activity to parents and carers, and suggest that they take their children to woods and parks to follow paths.

*Physical development*

# Crossing the road

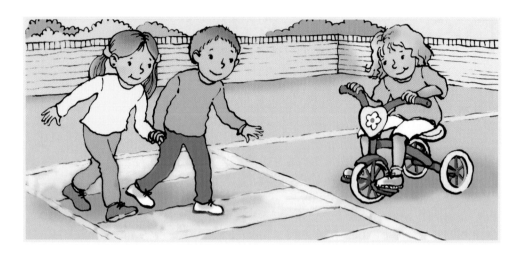

**Stepping Stone**
Negotiate an appropriate pathway when walking, running or using a wheelchair or other mobility aids, both indoors and outdoors.

**Early Learning Goal**
Show awareness of space, of themselves and of others.

■

**Group size**
Eight children.

■

**What you need**
Outdoor area; wheeled toy vehicles such as cars, bikes and trolleys; thick chalk.

■

**Preparation**
Create some tracks from chalk as in the activity 'Drive carefully!' on page 31, and incorporate any existing painted markings. Include pedestrian crossing points.

**Home links**
Explain the activity to parents and carers and ask them to show their children how to use pelican and zebra crossings.

## What to do
■ Take the children outdoors and show them the tracks that you have created. Ask them to tell you where they could cross the track safely if they were pedestrians.

■ Find a safe place to cross together and invite the children to take turns to cross the track safely with you, while the other children pretend to be the traffic. Introduce rules about holding an adult's hand and standing still on the pavement until the traffic stops before crossing a road.

■ Invite four of the children to ride bikes and cars along the marked tracks, while the other four children take the role of two adults and two children walking alongside.

■ Suggest that the pedestrians find safe places to cross the track, reminding them that the children must hold the hands of the adults.

■ Let younger children play the part of the children crossing the road with an adult to emphasise the importance of this safety rule.

■ Invite older children to play the part of adults to develop their confidence and encourage them to consider the needs of others.

## More ideas
■ Invite a road safety officer to visit your setting to explain basic safety rules, such as road signs and a pelican crossing, to the children. Ask them to loan equipment for the children to investigate.

■ Suggest that some children push dolls in buggies and cross the track safely with them.

## Other curriculum areas

PSED Play 'Stations'. Encourage the children to run along the tracks and choose the nearest station to stop at when you blow a whistle or hold up a red flag.

MD Invite the children to hold on to one another to form trains of different lengths with varying numbers of passengers.

# The lost rabbit

## What to do

■ Read the story 'Where is my burrow?' on the photocopiable sheet to the children. Talk about the characters and their movements.

■ Suggest to the children that they dramatise the story, and ask them which characters they would like to play. Allocate the different parts, and if several children choose the same one, explain that you will act out the story several times so that they can each have a turn to play a particular character.

■ Encourage the children to demonstrate appropriate movements for the animals that they represent, for example, the mole shuffling out of the plastic tunnel, the frog jumping in and out of 'lily pad' hoops, the hedgehog rolling around on the safety mat, and the mother rabbit hopping about outside the pop-up tent 'burrow'.

■ Re-enact the story as a whole group with younger children who may become restless while waiting for a turn to take part. They may enjoy just sitting down and watching older children re-enact the story at first, perhaps joining in with repeated phrases in the story.

■ Develop the self-confidence of older children by inviting them to perform the story in front of younger children or parents and carers.

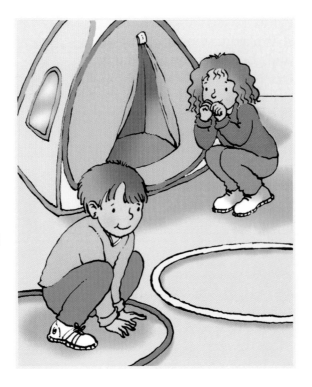

**Stepping Stone**
Judge body space in relation to spaces available when fitting into confined spaces or negotiating holes and boundaries.

**Early Learning Goal**
Show awareness of space, of themselves and of others.
■
**Group size**
Five children.
■
**What you need**
The photocopiable sheet 'Where is my burrow?' on page 85; plastic tunnel; four hoops; safety mat; pop-up tent.
■
**Preparation**
Arrange the apparatus in appropriate positions to represent the route taken by the rabbit in the story on the photocopiable sheet.

## More ideas

■ Provide opportunities for hiding in confined spaces and crawling through narrow boundaries, by using large recyclable boxes and fabric to create exciting imaginary landscapes such as the moon's surface.

■ Make caves, igloos, dens and other unusual homes with pop-up tents for varied role-play opportunities.

## Other curriculum areas

MD Introduce the children to appropriate mathematical language associated with size and position by re-enacting the story with plastic animals and recyclable materials.

CD Use recyclable materials, paints, glue and sticky tape to make models of the route taken by the rabbit in the story.

**Home links**
Give each child a copy of the photocopiable sheet to take home and suggest to parents and carers that they encourage their children to pretend to be the characters in the story, negotiating obstacles within their home or garden.

**Physical development**

# Clever messengers

**Early Learning Goal**
Show awareness of space, of themselves and of others.
∎

**Group size**
Six children to draw the plan; individual children to take messages.
∎

**What you need**
Large sheet of card; felt-tipped pens; black marker pen; glue; coloured paper; scissors.

## What to do
∎ Explain to the children that you would like one of them to take a message to another adult at the other side of the room. Talk about what the word 'message' means.
∎ Discuss the route that the child will take to deliver the message. Will it be possible to walk in a straight line? Why not?
∎ Suggest that you draw a plan of the room to show the children's position and that of the adult receiving the message. Represent obstacles by drawing outlines or sticking cut-out pieces of coloured paper on to the plan.

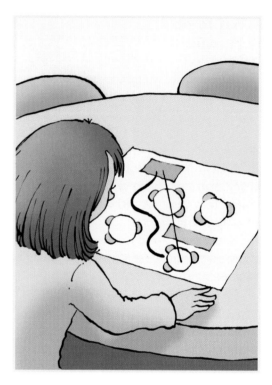

∎ Draw a straight line across the plan from the children's position to the adult. Note where the line crosses any obstacles.
∎ Invite a child to deliver the message and return. Talk about the route taken and draw this on the plan using a thick black pen, pointing to obstacles negotiated on the way.
∎ Let younger children simply deliver a message together and talk about the route that they have taken.
∎ Supply clipboards and encourage older children to draw their own plans and pictures of the routes taken when delivering the messages.

## More ideas
∎ Compare routes that are taken by air, rail and road. Which ones travel in straight lines? Which ones involve negotiating objects on the way? Why did carrier pigeons take messages?
∎ Make journeys with small-world vehicles across wet sand, involving negotiating hills and travelling through tunnels.

### Other curriculum areas
MD — Decide whether it is a shorter journey to travel along a straight line or a wavy line. Create straight and curved tracks between two points using small-world railway lines, and measure them with pieces of string.

KUW — Make a short journey, for example, to a local shop, and return by a different route. Compare what you see and discuss which route you all preferred.

**Home links**
Suggest that parents and carers involve their children in carrying out small tasks at home, involving following a chosen route, for example, going to post a letter.

**Physical development**

# Find a space

## What to do

▓ Stand with the children in the middle of a clear space and ask them if they can touch another person by stretching out their arms.

▓ Explain to the children that you would like them to have a space of their own so that they do not bump into anyone else while they dance to the music that you are going to play.

▓ Play some music and invite the children to find a space of their own when the music stops. Demonstrate how to stand with your arms spread wide and to turn around in a circle to make sure that your are not within touching distance of anyone else.

▓ Ask the children to follow simple directions, such as touching the floor and hopping, within their own space.

▓ Continue dancing to the music and find a space when the music stops, so that the children become more aware of the space around them.

▓ Carry out the activity with fewer younger children.

▓ Invite older children to dance to the music in pairs, avoiding other couples as they move around the floor, and sitting in a space of their own, as a pair, when the music stops.

## More ideas

▓ Play games such as 'Musical statues' or 'Musical bumps', dancing to music, then standing very still or sitting down quickly when the music stops.

▓ Spread some cushions on the floor and suggest to the children that they dance among them, without standing on them, then find a cushion of their own to sit on when the music stops.

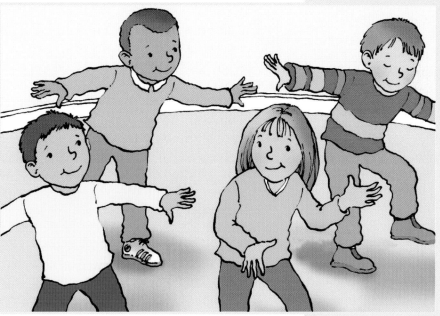

### Stepping Stone
Show respect for other children's personal space when playing among them.

### Early Learning Goal
Show awareness of space, of themselves and of others.

■

### Group size
Up to ten children.

■

### What you need
CD player or tape recorder; music CD or tape.

## Other curriculum areas

CD  Sing action songs such as 'Here We Go Round the Mulberry Bush' (Traditional) to encourage the children to move imaginatively alongside others.

MD  Build towers a safe distance away from one another using large bricks. Count the finished towers to see how many bricks are in each one.

### Home links
Suggest to parents and carers that they take their children to play among other children, for example, on large apparatus at a park, at a soft-play centre or in a swimming-pool.

# Knock them flat!

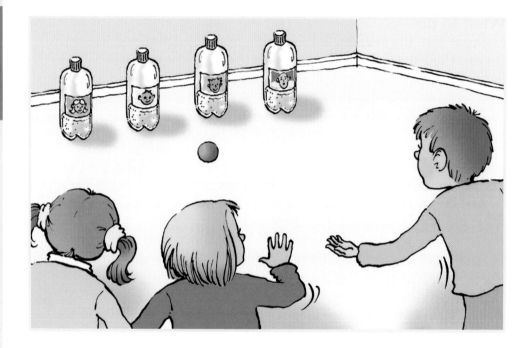

## What to do

■ Explain to the children that you are going to use the bottles to make a 'Skittles' game.

■ Ask each child to pour some rice or sand into the bottom of a bottle using a scoop and a funnel so that the bottle is more stable. Invite them to choose one of the card faces and colour it with felt-tipped pens before attaching it to the bottle with tape.

■ Demonstrate how to stand a finished skittle in the middle of a clear floor space and roll a ball at it to try to knock it over.

■ Explain to the children that the aim of the game is to knock over their own skittles without knocking over anybody else's.

■ Decide how far apart the skittles should be and how far away the children should stand.

■ For younger children, use larger balls and arrange the skittles close together. Suggest that they try to knock any of the skittles over rather than a specific one.

■ Invite older children to take turns to try to knock over as many skittles as they can before a sand-timer runs out.

## Other curriculum areas

MD ■ Play 'Ten-pin bowling' using the skittles and keep a tally of the number of skittles knocked over.

KUW ■ Roll balls down slopes and predict whether they will roll further and faster when the gradient is changed.

## More ideas

■ Invite the children to try to kick or roll a large sponge ball backwards and forwards to a friend across a clear floor space.

■ Suggest that half of the children hold hands and stand still with their legs apart while the other half try to roll large soft balls under the 'arches of the bridge' made by the first half.

# Follow the rules

## What to do

■ Explain to the children that you are concerned that some of them in the group might not be using apparatus safely and that you are going to write down what they need to remember.

■ Introduce the word 'rules' and read the rules on the photocopiable sheet to the children. Do all of these rules apply to using your apparatus? Can the children think of any to add? Write down their ideas, for example, taking turns on the slide. Explain your reasons for limiting the number of children using a piece of apparatus at any one time.

■ Invite the children to explore the apparatus, taking into account the rules that they have made.

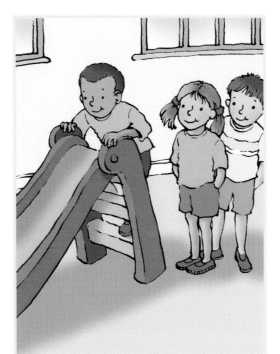

■ Afterwards, talk about the rules that the children followed as they used the equipment.

■ Type and print out a final choice of rules and display it near to the large apparatus area.

■ Ensure that apparatus for younger children is appropriate to their physical ability, and reinforce simple safety rules by explaining them while they are actually using the equipment.

■ Invite older children to consider the safety aspects of using outdoor apparatus, and let them be involved when creating a list of rules for outdoor play.

## More ideas

■ Encourage the children to devise appropriate rules for their own made-up games.

■ Involve the children in clearing away large and small apparatus safely by delegating tasks to small groups.

### Other curriculum areas

PSED  Encourage the children to devise their own rules for appropriate behaviour in indoor play areas, such as the sand area.

MD  Play games together that involve following a sequence of actions and counting and recognising numbers, for example, 'Snakes and ladders'.

**Stepping Stone**
Collaborate in devising and sharing tasks, including those which involve accepting rules.

Early Learning Goal
Show awareness of space, of themselves and of others.

■

Group size
Four children.

■

What you need
The photocopiable sheet 'Our rules' on page 87; sheet of white A4 card; clipboard with paper attached; felt-tipped pen; selection of large apparatus, including a slide and climbing frame.

■

Preparation
Set out the large apparatus before the activity and make a copy of the photocopiable sheet.

Home links
Suggest to parents and carers that they make up games with their children using balls and everyday items, for example, rolling a ball down a tray into a bucket.

# Tidy-up time!

Collaborate in devising and sharing tasks, including those which involve accepting rules.

**Early Learning Goal**
Show awareness of space, of themselves and of others.

■

**Group size**
Six children.

■

**What you need**
Tape recorder or CD player; music tape or CD; hand bell; three plastic storage containers with lids; beanbags; balls; quoits; three squares of card, approximately 25cm x 25cm; early years catalogue; black felt-tipped pen.

■

**Preparation**
Make labels for the containers by cutting out pictures of beanbags, balls and quoits from a catalogue. Glue a picture of each of the three types of small apparatus to a different square of card and write the name underneath. Attach each square to a storage container and fill the container with the appropriate apparatus.

## What to do
■ Place the storage containers on the floor with the lids on and invite the children to guess what is in them by looking at the labels. Remove the lids so that the children can explore the contents freely.

■ Explain to the children that you would like them to tidy up when they have finished playing. Invite them to choose a friend, so that there are three pairs of children, to tidy up, and allocate one type of apparatus to each pair.

■ Ask the children to suggest ways of indicating when it is time to tidy up, for example, ringing a bell or playing some music. Which signal would they like to use?

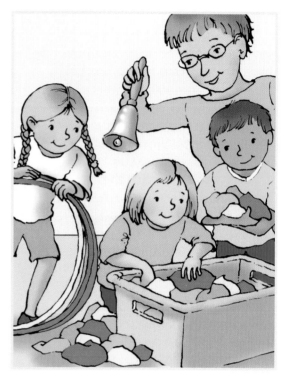

■ Suggest to the children that they carry on playing until they hear the signal to tidy up. They should then pick up their chosen apparatus and put it in the correct container.

■ Let younger children tidy up just one type of apparatus on a given signal.

■ Encourage older children to tidy different play areas in small groups, returning equipment to the designated places.

## More ideas
■ Ask the children to work in small groups to help with cleaning equipment, washing toys and cleaning work surfaces.

■ Invite small groups of children to choose resources to put out on a table and arrange them attractively for others to see.

**Home links**
Suggest to parents and carers that they involve their children in daily routines at home such as preparing food and setting the table.

## Other curriculum areas
PSED Encourage each child to manage their own snack time by setting out their snack and clearing away afterwards for the next child.

MD Devise storage systems that involve sorting, counting and matching different types of equipment.

# Forest camp

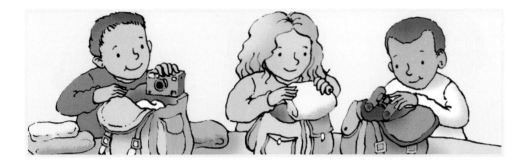

## What to do

■ Look together at the books, photographs and pictures of families camping. Talk to the children about camping holidays and invite them to share any experiences.

■ Show the children the collection of cartons, blankets and planks. Tell them that you would like to pretend to go on a camping expedition but that you have no real tents. Suggest that they make their own campsite from the resources.

■ Invite the children to try out their ideas. Decide whether you will build one big structure or several individual ones. Encourage different movements such as stretching, lying down and curling up as the children move the resources around.

■ When the living quarters are completed, return to the home area and ask the children what they think they will need for their holiday. Pack the rucksacks with clothes, food and utensils and ensure that additional items, such as the camera, binoculars and torch, are easily accessible.

■ Allow time for the children to play freely and encourage them to leave the site set up for other children to use afterwards.

■ Set up the campsite beforehand for younger children so that they can enjoy simply playing with the resources that are available.

■ Encourage older children to make up and dramatise their own camping stories.

## More ideas

■ Change the purpose of the building to link with a different theme, for example, a seaside hut, cave or castle.

■ Create a tepee using bamboo canes, tape and white sheeting, and paint the outside with appropriate designs.

### Other curriculum areas

PSED  Sukkot, the Jewish festival of Tabernacles, is celebrated each year during October. Create a sukkah from a pop-up tent covered with a sheet printed with fruit shapes.

CLL  Make up a book about an imaginary camping expedition in a forest, illustrated by the children, with captions written by adults and older children.

# What can you do?

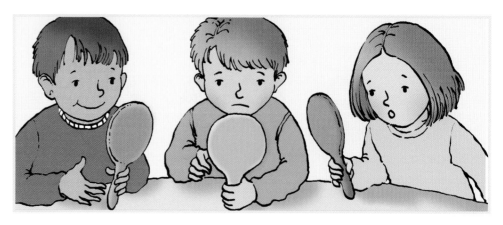

## What to do

◾ Draw the children's attention to their bodily movements by inviting them to take turns to stand in front of a full-length mirror and watch themselves as they move different limbs.

◾ Arrange smaller mirrors on a table and invite the children to observe their faces closely. Can they change their expressions so that they look pleased, unhappy, surprised or angry?

◾ Suggest that the children stand in pairs, facing each other. Ask one child in each pair to pretend to be a mirror and to copy the actions of the other child.

◾ Let younger children follow the actions of an adult, perhaps while singing an action rhyme, such as 'Heads and Shoulders, Knees and Toes' from *This Little Puffin...* compiled by Elizabeth Matterson (Puffin Books).

◾ Play 'Follow-my-leader' with older children. Ask adults to take turns with the children to play the part of the leader so that they can extend the range of movements.

## More ideas

◾ Play a simple form of charades and ask the children to mime everyday actions, such as washing hands or eating a meal.

◾ Pretend to move like different creatures, for example, walking on four legs like a horse, jumping on two legs like a kangaroo, flapping wings like a bird or sliding along the ground like a worm.

## Other curriculum areas

MD   Ask the children to move into different positions by including appropriate positional language in your instructions, such as 'high', 'low', 'over', 'under' and 'beside'.

CLL   Encourage the children to make verbal comparisons and extend their vocabulary by describing the movements that they make as they look into the mirrors, for example, 'as thin as a pin', 'as tiny as a mouse' and 'as tall as a giant'.

# Standing in a queue

## What to do

■ Talk to the children about travelling on a bus. Have they ever waited at a bus stop? Did they stand in a queue? Can they remember any other occasions when they have had to queue for something?

■ Invite the children to take a piece of card from the centre of the table, and explain about the sign that you have drawn. Are there any people queuing for a bus already?

■ Look through the catalogues to find pictures of adults and children, and invite each child to choose who they would like to have queuing at the bus stop on their piece of card.

■ Suggest that the children each cut out the pictures of their chosen people and stick them on to their card to form a picture of a bus queue.

■ Observe the children as they cut and emphasise how to use the scissors correctly. Ensure that any children who are left-handed have the option of using left-handed scissors.

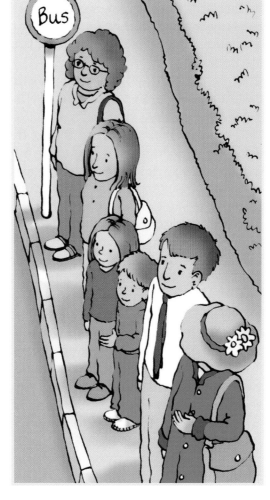

■ Present younger children with individual pages from the catalogues so that they can manage to cut or tear around the people that they have chosen more easily.

■ Challenge older children to cut out figures of different heights and to arrange them in order from the tallest to the shortest.

## More ideas

■ Thread beads on to laces to create regular patterns.

■ Punch holes around the outline of a definite shape, such as a fish, and invite the children to thread laces, wool or ribbon in and out of the holes.

### Other curriculum areas

**CLL** Encourage the children to develop up-and-down and circular letter movements when painting and drawing.

**CD** Invite the children to paint with large brushes on long rolls of wallpaper outdoors.

**Stepping Stone**
Show a clear and consistent preference for the left or right hand.

**Early Learning Goal**
Show awareness of space, of themselves and of others.

■

**Group size**
Six children.

■

**What you need**
Mail-order catalogues; right- and left-handed scissors; card; glue; spreaders; table

■

**Preparation**
Cut the card into rectangles and draw a bus-stop sign at one end of each piece of card. Place all the cards in the centre of the table.

**Home links**
Explain the learning objective to parents and carers so that they provide further opportunities for their children to enjoy activities to develop manual skills, such as cutting and sticking, at home.

**Physical development**

# Wriggling snakes

**Early Learning Goal**
Show awareness of space, of themselves and of others.

**Group size**
Six children.

**What you need**
Pictures of snakes; pasta tubes; paint in various colours; paintrushes; six lengths of string (approximately 60cm); artificial grass.

**Preparation**
Tie a pasta tube to the end of each length of string to prevent the rest of the tubes from falling off as the children make their snakes.

**Home links**
Send home instructions for making pasta necklaces, dough snakes and cotton-reel puppets.

## What to do
■ Show the children the pictures of snakes and suggest that they make some wriggling snakes of their own to pull along the floor.
■ Invite the children to paint a selection of pasta tubes in colours of their choice and allow them to dry.
■ Show the children how to thread the tubes on to a length of string to form a wriggling snake. Encourage them to look again at the pictures when considering patterns and how many different colours they want to use. Thread the string through the last tube twice and tie it so that it does not slip off.
■ Invite the children to pull their snakes along the floor, wriggling them as they do so. Display them on some artificial grass.
■ Fasten the string to a paper clip to make threading easier for younger children.
■ Let older children thread a variety of interesting objects on to string to form a necklace, for example, milk-bottle tops, buttons, tubes made from rolled paper, cut-up straws and cotton reels.

## More ideas
■ Make a caterpillar puppet by threading cotton reels through a length of string and tying them to a cane at each end and in the middle. The children can then shake the cane to make the caterpillar dance.
■ Create wriggling snakes from dough, and print patterns along them with different objects such as keys and pens.

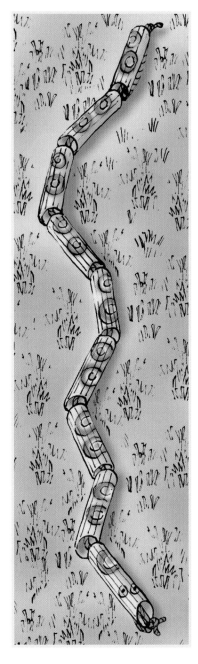

## Other curriculum areas
MD Draw faces on the ends of ten cotton reels and arrange them on a shoebox in a row. Sing the rhyme 'Ten in the Bed' from *This Little Puffin...* compiled by Elizabeth Matterson (Puffin Books) and roll a cotton reel off the box at the end of each verse.

KUW Encourage the children to mix their own dough to create the snakes and talk about changes as the ingredients are mixed.

### Chapter 3

The activities in this chapter concentrate on encouraging the children to begin to recognise the importance of keeping healthy and those things which contribute to this, and to recognise changes that happen to their bodies when they are active.

# Along the right lines

## What to do
■ Show the children the photographs of their regular routines and discuss what is happening in the photographs. Make links to keeping healthy when appropriate.

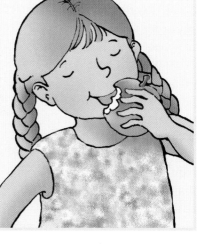

■ Ask a small group of children to arrange the photographs in order according to when they occur during a session, and to glue the photographs to a long strip of card in the order that they have decided.
■ Discuss what should be written underneath each photograph to describe the routine.
■ Attach the strip of card to a display board at child height and screw a plastic-coated cup hook to each end.
■ Thread a piece of string through a cotton reel and tie the string firmly to the cup hook at each end of the strip of card.
■ Encourage the children to move the cotton reel along as each routine is completed.
■ Discuss the importance of health routines with younger children while they are actually taking part in them, rather than talking about the photographs.
■ Encourage older children to write their own words to put underneath the photographs.

## More ideas
■ Have a 'routine shelf' with appropriate resources displayed along it representing the routines, such as a photocopied page from the register, cup, towel and hat for outdoors. Move a teddy along the shelf as the session progresses.
■ Introduce sound indicators for different routines, for example, beat a drum to signify 'tidy-up time'.

## Other curriculum areas
**MD** Use sand-timers to indicate how long the children can play before they need to tidy up.
**PSED** Create a 'helpers' rota' for older children, for example, helping to prepare snacks or assisting younger children with fastening coats.

**Stepping Stone**
Show awareness of own needs with regard to eating, sleeping and hygiene.

**Early Learning Goal**
Recognise the importance of keeping healthy and those things which contribute to this.

**Group size**
Up to 12 children for the discussion; up to four children to set up the line.

**What you need**
Photographs of regular routines such as registration, hand-washing, toilet-visiting, outdoor exercise, snacks and meals; display board; strip of card; scissors; thick felt-tipped pens; string; cotton reel; plastic-coated cup hook.

**Home links**
Encourage parents and carers to realise the importance of your daily routines by sending home a sheet explaining some of the learning objectives for each one.

# No more germs

**Early Learning Goal**
Recognise the importance of keeping healthy and those things which contribute to this.

**Group size**
Six children.

**What you need**
Access to hand-washing facilities, including soap and towels.

## What to do
■ Towards the end of a session, ask the children to talk about when they have washed their hands during the session. What were the reasons for washing them? Discuss how washing hands removes dirt and germs and prevents the children from becoming ill.

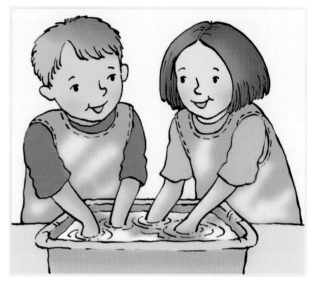

■ Encourage the children to think about the different movements that they use when washing their hands. What do they do first? What is the last thing that they do?
■ Sing 'Here We Go Round the Mulberry Bush' (Traditional), then make up a verse for each hand-washing action. Carry out actions such as 'This is the way we roll up our sleeves', 'turn on the tap', 'put on the soap', 'rub our hands together', 'rinse off the soap', 'dry our hands' and, finally, 'throw away the paper towel'.
■ Visit the cloakroom or hand-washing bowl and invite the children to take turns to wash their hands. Talk together about the actions as they carry them out.
■ Examine the children's clean hands and praise them for their actions.
■ Demonstrate each stage of hand-washing to younger children and help them if their hands are very soiled.
■ Encourage older children to support younger children, for example, helping them to roll up their sleeves and turn off the taps.

## More ideas
■ Make some laminated signs to remind the children to wash their hands. Invite older children to illustrate them.
■ Bath some dolls and use the activity to stimulate discussion about the importance of bathtime routines.

**Home links**
Send home copies of your made-up song about hand-washing and encourage parents and carers to sing it with their children at home.

## Other curriculum areas
KUW Put some blobs of paint on a doll and allow them to dry before trying to wash them off in different conditions, for example, in cold or warm water, and with or without soap. Discuss the most effective materials for removing dirt and stains.

CLL Sing 'Here We Go Round the Mulberry Bush' and include verses about washing hair and cleaning teeth.

# Time for bed

## What to do

■ Talk about the newly created bedroom and make comparisons with the children's own bedrooms.

■ Discuss the children's home bedtime routines, remembering to include different cultural practices as appropriate, and explain to the children the importance of sleep.

■ Play with the children in the bedroom area, acting out the routine of getting ready for bed. Explain that sharing brushes, towels and washing materials would not be hygienic and suggest that the children mime the actions of cleaning their teeth, washing and brushing their hair instead. Tell the children that there is no need to undress, as this is just pretend. Encourage them children to put the night-clothes over their own clothes.

■ Invite each child to get into a bed.

■ Read one of the bedtime stories to the children, then leave them to play by themselves.

■ Talk to younger children about each action, emphasising that the play is just 'pretend'.

■ Encourage older children to take turns to be the adult and read the bedtime stories.

## More ideas

■ Use dolls' beds and clothes, rather than child-size, and prepare the dolls for bed.

■ Re-enact the routines associated with getting up in the morning in the home area and include breakfast time.

### Home links

Invite parents and carers to talk through bedtime routines with their children and encourage them to choose favourite stories to read.

### Other curriculum areas

KUW — Invite the children to draw pictures of their experiences of day and night.

CLL — Ask the children to choose their favourite bedtime story-books and make a display with illustrations and captions.

### Stepping Stone

Show awareness of a range of healthy practices with regard to eating, sleeping and hygiene.

### Early Learning Goal

Recognise the importance of keeping healthy and those things which contribute to this.

### Group size

Two children.

### What you need

Two children's beds or sleep mats; pillows; blankets; two teddy bears; books of bedtime stories; small table; toy night-light; large night-clothes to fit over the children's own clothes; slippers; black paper; silver foil; scrap fabric; masking tape; storage box.

### Preparation

Transform the home area into a bedroom. Create a 'window' on the wall with black paper and a silver-foil moon. Add some curtains made from scrap fabric, attached to either side of the 'window' with masking tape. Arrange the other resources appropriately.

*Physical development*

# Snack time

**Stepping Stone**
Show awareness of a range of healthy practices with regard to eating, sleeping and hygiene.

**Early Learning Goal**
Recognise the importance of keeping healthy and those things which contribute to this.

**Group size**
Four children for the preparation; whole group for eating.

**What you need**
Soft spread; sliced white and brown bread; plastic knives; selection of fruit; chopping boards; large bowl; small bowls; large plate; small plates; paper towels; spoons.

**Preparation**
Check for any food allergies and dietary requirements.

**Home links**
Obtain a selection of leaflets on healthy eating, available from your local health department, to send home to parents and carers, encouraging them to promote this with their children.

## What to do
■ Invite the children to help you prepare a snack for the rest of the group.
■ Give each child a chopping board and ask them to cut the pieces of fruit into smaller portions, and put them into the large bowl. Explain that eating fruit is part of a healthy diet.
■ Give each child a slice of bread to cover with soft spread and cut into quarters. Put the cut-up pieces of bread on to a large plate. Talk about the importance of eating a good range of foods in order to keep healthy.

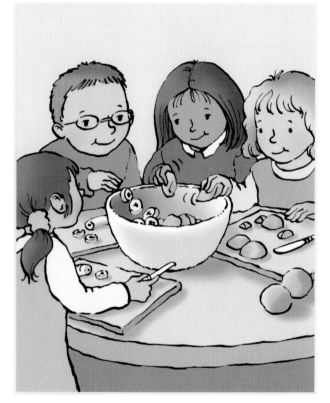

■ Decide together how many tables to set. Share out the fruit and bread so that there is a plate of bread and a bowl of fruit for each table.
■ Invite the children to set a place for each child in your setting with a plate, bowl, spoon and paper towel, and to put a bowl and plate of prepared food in the centre of each table.
■ When the other children have taken their places, introduce the four children who have helped and ask them to tell the others what they did. Talk about the importance of healthy eating together.
■ Give younger children softer fruit to cut up, such as bananas, melon and peaches.
■ Invite older children to prepare some stewed fruit, such as apples or rhubarb, and serve this warm on a cold day.

## More ideas
■ Make observational drawings of different vegetables, and have tasting sessions to compare raw and cooked vegetables.
■ Talk about the importance of milk for healthy teeth and bones. Prepare and taste dishes such as milk puddings and blancmange.

### Other curriculum areas
**PSED** Prepare and taste foods from other cultures, using appropriate utensils, such as a wok, chopsticks and rice bowls.
**MD** Taste a range of different breakfast cereals and make a block graph to indicate the children's favourites.

**Physical development**

# Making choices

## What to do
■ Talk to the children about feeling thirsty and hungry, and why we need to have drinks, snacks and meals.
■ Discuss the importance of eating a balanced selection of foods, including fruit, vegetables, bread, rice, pasta and potatoes.

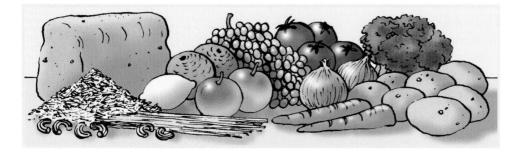

■ Suggest that the children prepare a snack menu for the following week.
■ Spread the days of the week cards in a row along a table. Show the children the pictures of snack foods and ask them to choose a snack for each day. Arrange the chosen pictures on the cards.
■ Talk about their choices and make modifications after discussion, for example, if there are too many sweet snacks, or days without fruit.
■ Discuss appropriate drinks and write down the children's choice for each day on a cup-shaped card. Explain how sugary drinks can cause tooth decay.
■ Stick the pictures of foods and drinks on to the sheet of A3 card, arranged in order from Monday to Friday.
■ Rather than involve younger children in the preparation of the menu card, refer to it as they eat their snacks and talk about the different foods that they are enjoying.
■ Involve older children as much as possible when planning for snack time, for example, by shopping together for foods.

## More ideas
■ Have theme weeks relating to festivals, with foods from the different cultures discussed.
■ Grow mustard and cress seedlings to add flavour to sandwiches.

## Other curriculum areas
CLL Set up a role-play café and encourage the children to include a good variety of food in their menus.
KUW Make some toast and talk about the changes as the bread browns.

### Home links
Display the menu cards for parents and carers to see, and encourage them to talk about them with their children.

# Caring for teeth

## What to do
■ Look at the pictures of the smiling faces and ask the children to smile at one another to show off their teeth.

■ Ask the children if they know what they can do to keep their teeth clean and sparkling. Refer to the activity 'Making choices' on page 47 about not eating too many sugary foods that would stick to their teeth. Explain the word 'decay' and talk about when the children clean their teeth and why.

■ Invite the children to take turns to pull something out of the drawstring bag and talk about it. Put the items on the floor and arrange them in the order that they are used when cleaning teeth.

■ Talk through the process of cleaning teeth, holding up the items as you do so.

■ Put a small toothbrush, a toothpaste box and a mug into the home area so that younger children can pretend to clean the dolls' teeth. Emphasise that they should not put the brush into their own mouths.

■ Encourage older children to take turns to talk to the rest of the group about when and how they clean their teeth, putting the actions into the correct sequence.

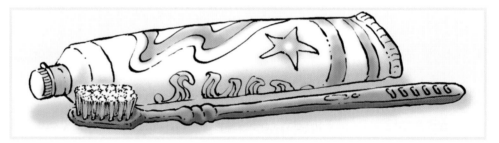

## More ideas
■ Invite a dentist or dental hygienist to visit your setting to talk to the children about dental care.

■ Copy the photocopiable sheet 'Regular routines' on page 88 on to card and cut out the pictures. Talk about the different objects and the routines that they are associated with. Challenge the children to arrange them in matching pairs.

## Other curriculum areas
CD Give each child a large tooth made from white card and a new toothbrush to brush it with white paint. (Do not use old toothbrushes as these could carry germs.) Talk about correct brushing movements as you do so.

MD Make a graph of favourite toothbrush colours using coloured card cut into a toothbrush shape.

# Warm or cold?

## What to do

■ Discuss what the children are wearing at the moment and how clothes vary in different weathers.

■ Sit in a circle around the clothes container and invite a child to choose something suitable to wear on a hot day. Talk about their choice.

■ Let the children take turns to find other clothes to wear, for example, on cold, wet or windy days. Encourage them to tell everyone the reasons for their choices.

■ Draw around one of the children on a length of wallpaper. Cut out the outline and stick it to one half of the wall display. Repeat with the other half of the display.

■ Dress the outline on the light-blue paper by stapling suitable clothes for a hot day. Contrast this by dressing the other outline in clothing for a cold day.

■ Concentrate on the clothing that younger children are actually wearing on the day and dress one outline according to the present season rather than make contrasts. Name the articles of clothing.

■ Encourage older children to write labels for the display and create features for the outlines using scraps of fabric.

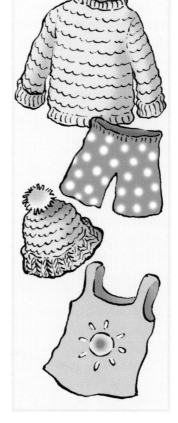

## More ideas

■ Make a copy of the photocopiable sheet 'Dressed for the weather' on page 89 on to card for each child. Cut the sheet in half and cut out the pictures. Give each child an outline of the figure together with their pictures, and ask them to choose appropriate clothes to wear in warm and cold weather.

■ Pack two suitcases, one for a holiday in a hot country and one for a visit to a very cold land.

## Other curriculum areas

**KUW** Talk about how clothes insulate the body against cold weather. Conduct simple investigations by wrapping up plastic bottles full of warm water in various materials and comparing how long they take to cool.

**MD** Count gloves, mittens and shoes, and sort them into matching pairs.

**Stepping Stone**
Show some understanding that good practices with regard to exercise, eating, sleeping and hygiene can contribute to good health.

**Early Learning Goal**
Recognise the importance of keeping healthy and those things which contribute to this.

■

**Group size**
Six children.

■

**What you need**
Selection of clothing suitable for warm and cold weather, for example, shorts, sandals, woollen jumper and scarf; storage container; light-blue and dark-blue frieze paper; length of white wallpaper; white paper; fabric scraps; pencil; scissors; glue; staple gun (adult use).

■

**Preparation**
Back a display board with frieze paper so that one half is light blue and the other is dark blue. Put the clothes into the storage container.

### Home links
Give each child a card copy of the photocopiable sheet to take home, and encourage parents and carers to complete it with their children.

# Pizza fun

## What to do
■ Talk with the children about their experiences of eating pizzas. Which toppings do they enjoy? Explain that pizzas are an ideal snack because of the variety of healthy ingredients.
■ Discuss why it is important to eat fresh vegetables, how cheese helps bones and teeth to grow strong, and how bread gives us energy.
■ Suggest to the children that they create their own 'muffin pizzas'. Give each child a muffin and a knife, and help them to cut the muffin in half.
■ Prepare the toppings together by grating the cheese and slicing the sausages, ham, mushrooms and peppers. Put the prepared ingredients into small individual bowls.
■ Encourage each child to chop up a small tomato into pieces and mix it in their bowl with a teaspoon of tomato purée to make a sauce and spread it on both of their bases.
■ Invite the children to choose freely from the toppings and arrange them on to the sauce before sprinkling grated cheese on top. Encourage them to think of their own ideas, such as creating funny faces.
■ Melt the cheese under a grill until it is bubbling, and leave the pizzas to cool slightly before letting the children eat them.
■ Limit the choice of toppings for younger children and help them with the preparation.
■ Encourage older children to invent toppings from a wider range of foods.

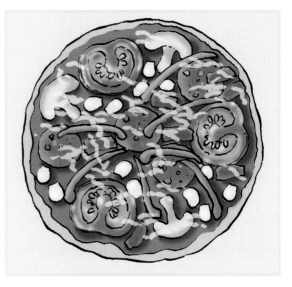

## More ideas
■ Make comparisons between different ways of eating potatoes, such as roast, mashed and jacket potatoes, chips and crisps.
■ Prepare different toppings for the pizzas, such as cottage cheese and pineapple or baked beans and tuna.

### Home links
Give each child a copy of the photocopiable sheet to take home. Encourage parents and carers to make the pizzas at home with their children.

### Other curriculum areas
KUW Sprinkle grated cheese over hot cooked pasta. Observe, touch and smell similarities and differences between raw and cooked pasta, and solid and melted cheese.
MD Count pieces of pasta and sort them by shape, colour and size.

# Vital organs

## What to do

■ Talk to the children about the function of the heart. Can they feel their hearts beating? Explain about the pumping action of the heart and see if they can locate a pulse in their wrists.

■ Ask the children to stand up and jump up and down as fast as they can. Do they notice any difference in the speed of their heartbeats?

■ Let the children rest for a few minutes, then talk about the way that the lungs work. Ask them to take some big breaths. Can they feel their chests moving in and out?

■ Encourage the children to jump up and down again. What do they notice about their breathing?

■ Invite a child to put on the tabard and ask another child to position the heart on the correct Velcro square. Do the other children agree with the position? Now ask another child to put the lungs in the correct place.

■ Rather than use the tabard, just talk to younger children about their hearts beating, and raise their awareness of their chests moving as they breathe in and out.

■ Let older children locate the position of other body parts and discover their functions.

## More ideas

■ Invite the children to watch themselves as they breathe in and out in front of a mirror.

■ Hang the tabard on a coat-hanger alongside a small table display of books and posters about the human body. Include paper and crayons and encourage children to explore the resources freely.

### Home links
Suggest to parents and carers that their children borrow library books about how the human body works.

### Other curriculum areas
KUW Talk about the function of muscles and consider the muscles that are used when playing football or throwing a ball.

CD Ask the children to paint pictures of physical activities that they enjoy.

### Stepping Stone
Observe the effects of activity on their bodies.

### Early Learning Goal
Recognise the changes that happen to their bodies when they are active.

■

### Group size
Six children.

■

### What you need
Red and pink fabric; cotton wool; large piece of fabric in a plain contrasting colour; needle (adult use); strong thread; Velcro; tape; scissors; tape measure.

■

### Preparation
Create a tabard with heart and lungs attached. Cut out a piece of plain fabric, hem it around the rough edges, and cut a hole for the head. Attach Velcro squares in appropriate positions for the lungs and heart (see diagram). Create heart and lungs by sewing pieces of red and pink fabric together and padding them with cotton wool.

# Beating hearts

**Stepping Stone**
Observe the effects of activity on their bodies.

**Early Learning Goal**
Recognise the changes that happen to their bodies when they are active.

**Group size**
Six children.

**What you need**
Stethoscope; drum; clear space.

## What to do

■ Show the children the stethoscope. Have they seen one before? Do they know what a stethoscope is used for? Can they tell the others about their experience?

■ Explain to the children how a stethoscope helps a doctor or nurse to listen to someone's heart beating, and invite the children to take turns to listen to each other's hearts.

■ Show the children how to locate their pulses and see if they can count ten beats.

■ Ask the children to stand very still, then when you beat a drum, to start running around in and out of one another until you stop beating the drum.

■ Invite the children to feel their pulses again. What do they notice? Ask them to count ten beats. Did they count faster than before?

■ Explain how vigorous exercise makes the heart beat faster and talk about the importance of regular exercise to keep us healthy. Take turns to use the stethoscope to listen to heartbeats before and after exercise.

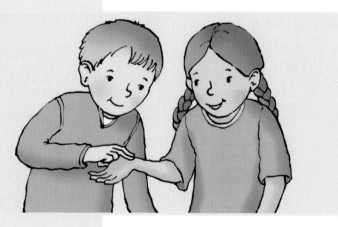

■ Do the children notice any other changes in their bodies? What happens to their breathing after exercise? Talk about being 'out of breath'.

■ Encourage younger children to run about, then stop and talk about being 'out of breath', rather than use the stethoscope and locate their pulses.

■ Ask older children to dance to fast music, then to lie still and listen to slow, dreamy music. Invite them to make comparisons between the effects on the body after vigorous exercise and after relaxation.

## More ideas

■ Play games that involve bursts of activity followed by a period of stillness, such as 'Musical statues'.

■ Encourage the children to enjoy periods of relaxation as part of your daily routine, for example, by listening to quiet music before snack time.

## Other curriculum areas

CLL   Set up a role-play doctor's surgery and include the stethoscope for the children to use.

PSED   Play vigorous ring games together, such as 'Ring-o-ring-o-Roses' and 'The Hokey Cokey' (Traditional).

**Home links**
Invite parents and carers to watch their children take part in physical 'fun' events at the end of the session, such as obstacle courses, and use this opportunity to explain the importance of regular exercise.

# Dressing for exercise

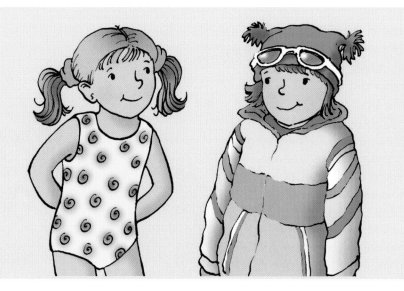

## What to do

■ Ask the children to run around in an open space and then to jump up and down on the spot. Do they feel warm or cool? What could they do to keep cooler during exercise? Invite them to take off their jumpers and cardigans. Does this make them feel cooler?

■ Talk about the importance of wearing appropriate clothing for exercise. Do the children have older brothers and sisters? What do they wear for physical activities and sports?

■ Show the children the examples of sportswear. Can they identify any of the sports from the items of clothing? Why do runners wear vests and shorts while skiers wear thick jackets and trousers?

■ With younger children, focus on the importance of dressing appropriately for exercise by helping them to remove their outer garments before physical activities and put them on again afterwards.

■ Encourage older children to take off their own outer clothing before exercise and dress themselves again afterwards.

## More ideas

■ Talk about the importance of warm-up and cool-down exercises and include them as part of your routine during physical activity.

■ Set up a role-play sportswear shop.

## Other curriculum areas

CD Look at catalogues showing sportswear and cut out some of the pictures to make collage scenes, for example, skiers in the snow or cyclists in a race.

MD Display appropriate protective footwear for different sports and ask the children to sort them into pairs.

### Stepping Stone
Observe the effects of activity on their bodies.

### Early Learning Goal
Recognise the changes that happen to their bodies when they are active.

### Group size
Six children.

### What you need
Open space; selection of sportswear such as a swimming costume and goggles, football strip and boots, running vest and shoes, and ski wear.

### Preparation
Send home a letter inviting parents and carers to loan sports equipment and clothing for a display.

### Home links
Invite parents and carers who regularly take part in a sport to come and talk to the children about what they do, and to demonstrate the clothing that they wear and equipment that they use.

# Let's relax

## Stepping Stone
Observe the effects of activity on their bodies.

## Early Learning Goal
Recognise the changes that happen to their bodies when they are active.

## Group size
Eight children.

## What you need
Open space; tape recorder or CD player; tapes or CDs of rousing music, such as 'Baba Yaga' from *Pictures at an Exhibition* by Mussorgsky, and relaxing music, such as 'Morning Mood' from the *Peer Gynt Suite* by Grieg.

## What to do
■ Ask the children to jump, run or hop around the room until they feel really tired, before sitting down. How did they know when they were tired?
■ Talk about feeling 'out of breath' after exercise. Invite the children to lie still for a few minutes and discuss what happens to their rate of breathing.
■ Play some rousing music to the children, followed by some relaxing music. Can they explain how the music makes them feel?
■ Invite the children to move freely to the rousing music and then to rest while you play the relaxing music. Discuss the effects of exercise and rest on the body, and emphasise how both are essential to a healthy lifestyle.

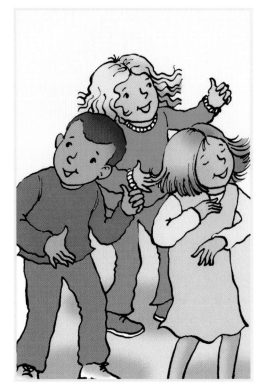

■ Play the rousing music to younger children and ask them to move freely before suggesting that they have a rest and listen to the relaxing music. Use vocabulary such as 'exercise', 'tired' and 'rest'.
■ Invite older children to choose their own music to dance to and then to relax to, and encourage them to talk about the changes that they notice in their bodies.

## More ideas
■ Play examples of recordings of solo instruments and invite the children to choose which instruments are suitable to listen to while they rest, for example, a quiet piano or a slow violin.
■ Encourage the children to close their eyes and imagine something that makes them feel happy and relaxed as they rest.

## Other curriculum areas
CD   Play relaxing music while the children are painting, then contrast this by playing rousing music. Does the choice of music affect the children's approach to their painting?

PSED   Use instruments from different cultures to create rousing and relaxing music. Invite the children to move freely to the sounds that they hear, for example, dancing rhythmically to African drums or relaxing to Indian bells.

## Home links
Encourage parents and carers to play soothing music to their children at bedtime to help them to feel secure and relaxed.

With this selection of activities, the children will learn how to use a variety of equipment. Suggested resources range from the usual large and small apparatus, such as climbing frames, slides and beanbags, to everyday items, such as blankets, cushions and boxes.

# Push or pull?

## What to do

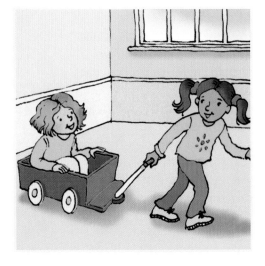

▮ Walk around the equipment together, stopping at each piece of equipment to talk about it. What is it called? How many wheels does it have?

▮ Invite a child to sit in a cart and ask another child to take them for a short ride. Encourage the rest of the group to watch.

▮ Talk about how the child made the cart move. Introduce the word 'pull'. What other things do the children pull along?

▮ Ask the children to find something to take a doll for a ride in. Stop them after a short while and ask how they made the equipment move. Introduce the word 'push'. What other things can be moved by pushing? Do the children enjoy being pushed on a swing?

▮ Invite the children to choose another piece of equipment and try to make it move. Stop after a short time to talk about the different movements that they have made.

▮ Use sit-and-ride cars, baby walkers and smaller tricycles for younger children.

▮ Challenge older children to use apparatus that requires co-operation, such as a tricycle with two seats.

## More ideas

▮ Invite the children to push a toy shopping trolley around a chalk-marked route. Attach a toy train to a piece of string and ask the children to pull it along the same route.

▮ Open and close a door. Which movement involves pushing and which involves pulling?

## Other curriculum areas

KUW Push an empty wheelbarrow around in your outdoor area, then fill it with sand. Is it easier or harder to push when it is full?

CD Make toy cars from recyclable materials and attach string to pull them along.

**Stepping Stone**
Operate equipment by means of pushing and pulling movements.

Early Learning Goal
Use a range of small and large equipment.
▮

Group size
Six children.
▮

What you need
Large hard-surfaced area; selection of wheeled equipment such as cars, bicycles, shopping trolleys, large pull-along carts, baby walkers, scooters, wheelbarrows, and dolls' prams and buggies; dolls.
▮

Preparation
Display the equipment on a hard surface.

Home links
Ask parents and carers to involve their children in pushing and pulling movements at home, for example, as they help to sweep the floor or hang up the washing.

# Cat in the well

**Early Learning Goal**
Use a range of small
and large equipment.
■
**Group size**
Four children.
■
**What you need**
A copy of the rhyme
'Ding Dong Bell'
(Traditional); small
and large bucket;
washing line; broom
handle; two chairs;
masking tape; soft
toy cat; cotton reel;
string.

## What to do
■ Sing the nursery rhyme 'Ding Dong Bell' and mime the actions of putting the cat in the well and pulling it out again. Emphasise to the children that this is not a true story and that we should never put a real cat in a well.

■ Suggest to the children that they make a model well. Push two chairs close together with their backs facing one another and put the large bucket on the floor between them to represent the well. Suspend a broom handle between the two chairs and tape the ends securely. Tie a cotton reel on a loop of string over the handle of the broom.

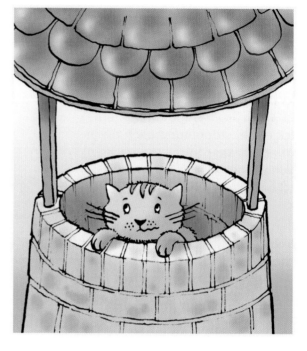

■ Tie the washing line to the small bucket, put the toy cat into it and lower it into the 'well'. Stretch the line through the loop of string, over the cotton reel.

■ Take turns to pull on the washing line to lift the bucket out of the well, as the rest of the group says the rhyme. Emphasise that this is 'pretend' and that it would be cruel to put a real cat into a bucket.

■ Encourage younger children to fill small buckets in the water tray and pull them out of the water by their handles.

■ Challenge older children to push different-shaped, partially blown balloon under some water.

## More ideas
■ Invite the children to ride scooters and talk about the pushing movements that are needed to make them go.

■ Sing 'See-saw Margery Daw' (Traditional) and ask two children to sit on a see-saw, talking about how it works.

## Other curriculum areas
PSED Invite the children to work with a partner. Ask them to sit on the floor, join hands to 'see-saw' backwards and forwards, and sing 'Row, Row, Row Your Boat' (Traditional).

MD Push small cars down ramps and measure how far they travel. Talk about the 'longest' and 'shortest' distances.

**Home links**
Suggest to parents
and carers that they
take their children to
a park so that they
can develop pushing
and pulling skills on
large climbing and
balancing
equipment.

**Physical development**

# Rolling along

## What to do
▓ Explain to the children that you want to create a slope to roll things down, similar to a slide. Try out the children's suggestions for making various slopes.

▓ Create several slopes of different lengths and heights with the planks and boxes.

▓ Invite the children to put the remaining resources at the top of the slopes, one by one, to see if they will move downwards. What happens when a wooden brick is put on a slope? Will it move if it is pushed? How steep does the gradient have to be before the brick will move without being pushed?

▓ Roll a small log down the slope. What happens if you put it upright on the slope?

▓ Which item rolls the fastest? Is it possible to roll something up a slope? Does the gradient of the slope affect the distance and speed that a log will roll?

▓ Set up three different slopes for younger children and give them lengths of dowelling to roll down the slopes.

▓ Invite older children to devise roller-coaster rides for small-world people in cars. Discuss how they need to push the cars to the top of the slopes so that they can roll down the other side.

## More ideas
▓ Sing 'Wind the Bobbin Up' from *This Little Puffin...* compiled by Elizabeth Matterson (Puffin Books) and encourage the children to make appropriate winding and pulling actions with their hands.

▓ Show the children how to operate a hand whisk to create bubbles in a bowl of water with washing-up liquid.

## Other curriculum areas
KUW  Invite the children to make simple kites with paper and string and run about outside on a windy day, pulling them behind them.

CD  Print patterns by pushing or pulling a paint roller across a sheet of paper. Are the finished patterns the same?

### Home links
Let the children make kites to take home and suggest to parents and carers that they fly them with their children and help them to wind the string in and out.

### Stepping Stone
Operate equipment by means of pushing and pulling movements.

### Early Learning Goal
Use a range of small and large equipment.
▓

### Group size
Four children.
▓

### What you need
Large space; various lengths of planks of wood; small logs; rolling-pins; cardboard tubes; wooden bricks; boxes of varying heights.

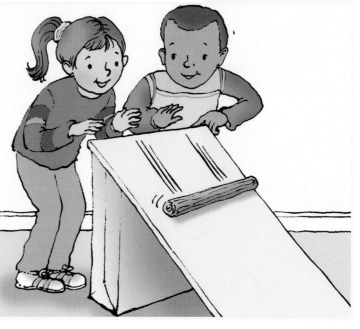

**Physical development**

# Wagon rides

**Early Learning Goal**
Use a range of small and large equipment.
■

**Group size**
Four children.
■

**What you need**
Two large pull-along carts.

## What to do

▧ Invite the children to work with a partner and to choose a pull-along cart to ride on.

▧ Suggest that one child sit in the cart while the other moves it. Talk about the best way to make the cart move. What is the purpose of the handle at the front?

▧ Let the children have free play with the carts and ensure that all the children have had a turn to pull and to ride the carts.

▧ Suggest that two children climb into one cart, one child climb into the other and the fourth child try to pull each one in turn. Which cart is the easiest to pull? Discuss the child's findings.

▧ Ask the children to get out of the carts, leave one empty and choose someone to climb back into the other. Take turns to pull the two carts and make comparisons.

▧ Try different combinations of pulling and pushing the carts, for example, two children riding, one pulling the handle and the other pushing from the back.

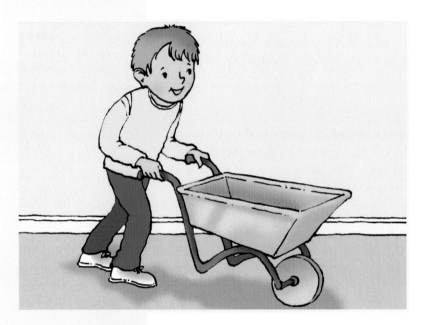

▧ Talk about the different muscles that are needed to pull and push the carts, and discuss which action the children find easiest.

▧ Let younger children just pull and push soft toys in buggies and small carts.

▧ Encourage older children to use carts and wheelbarrows to transport resources, for example, when building a den outdoors.

## More ideas

▧ Incorporate carts into role-play by using them as trains or buses for imaginary journeys.

▧ Ask the children to compare the pushing movements needed to move tricycles, for example, using their feet or pushing down the pedals. Which is easiest?

## Other curriculum areas

PSED Organise a sponsored 'push' with the children pushing dolls in toy prams and buggies around a given route, to raise money for charity.

MD Take dolls for rides in carts and focus on mathematical language to describe size, position and capacity, for example, 'bigger', 'smallest', 'in front', 'beside', 'full', 'empty' and so on.

**Home links**
Suggest to parents and carers that they encourage their children to help them push supermarket trolleys and talk about how they need to push harder as the trolley gets full.

# Let's move house!

## What to do

Read the story 'Maisy moves house' on the photocopiable sheet and talk to the children about their own experiences of moving house.

Suggest to the children that they build a new house on the floor using the resources on display.

Use the boxes and planks to form a frame, and drape curtains or blankets over it. Interact with the children, trying out their suggestions and extending their ideas.

Talk about the things that the children will need to bring from the home area to make their new creation feel like 'home'. Emphasise that they will have to carry things in suitcases, so large things will have to stay behind.

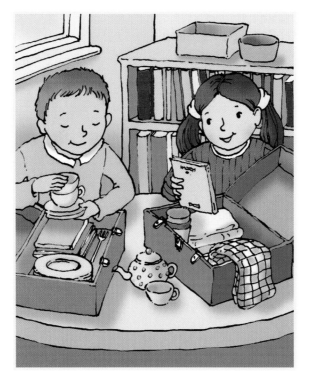

Go to the home area and work together to pack the suitcases. If there is sufficient floor space, pile the cases on a pull-along cart to represent a furniture van and pull it to the new home.

Allow time for the children to play freely in their new home.

Be sensitive to the fact that younger children might feel anxious enclosed in a dark space, and design the house with this in mind.

Challenge older children to include extras in their house, such as windows, doors and a garden, using recyclable materials.

## More ideas

Invite the children to create their own secret places, dens and homes outdoors. Encourage them to use any natural features, such as bushes and trees, to shelter under.

Construct fantasy homes, such as castles and caves, using climbing apparatus, tunnels and barrels.

## Other curriculum areas

CLL  Make a bridge from planks and boxes to dramatise the story of 'The Three Billy Goats Gruff' (Traditional).

MD  Use construction equipment to create separate houses for three bears of different sizes.

Stepping Stone
Construct with large materials such as cartons, long lengths of fabric and planks.

Early Learning Goal
Use a range of small and large equipment.

Group size
Four children.

What you need
The photocopiable sheet 'Maisy moves house' on page 91; clear floor space; large cardboard boxes; short lightweight planks; blankets, sheets or curtains; two small suitcases; resources from the home area; pull-along cart.

Preparation
Put the small suitcases in the home area and leave the house-building resources randomly in the centre of the space.

Home links
Send home a copy of the story on the photocopiable sheet and encourage parents and carers to build dens and tents with their children.

# Warm and cosy

## What to do

■ Talk to the children about how some creatures hibernate in the long, cold winter months. Explain that they keep warm and safe by creating cosy spaces where they can sleep without being disturbed.

■ Read the rhyme 'Secret places' on the photocopiable sheet to the children and talk about making cosy dens.

■ Invite the children to pretend to be a family of bears looking for a warm cave for their winter sleep.

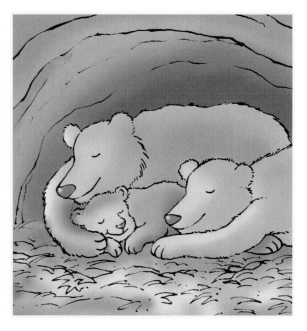

Walk around the room and stop in front of the resources. Suggest that this would be a good place if only there was a cave to curl up in. Could the children make a cave from the materials in front of them?

■ Work together to make the cave, then sit on the floor in front of the finished cave. Look inside and talk about whether the bears will be comfortable. Is there something to lie on?

■ Show the children the 'autumn' coloured paper and suggest that they tear it up into small leaves and spread them on the floor of the cave.

■ Allow time for the family of bears to play freely.

■ Help younger children to build the cave and be aware of possible safety issues when positioning the planks.

■ Discuss the importance of being hidden from other animals and ask older children to think of ways of disguising the cave, for example, by covering it with paper leaves and twigs.

## More ideas

■ Use a tunnel leading into a pop-up tent to make a rabbit's burrow. Disguise the structure with drapes of green fabric.

■ Encourage the children to arrange apparatus to form an imaginary landscape, then pretend to be dinosaurs travelling across it.

## Other curriculum areas

**KUW** Form a circle with cardboard boxes and imagine being birds building nests, filling them with soft cushions and fabric.

**CLL** Create a fantasy story cave with boxes and drapes and sit inside to share adventure stories.

# Pirate ship

## What to do

■ Sing the song 'Ahoy there!' on the photocopiable sheet and talk about the life of a pirate. Familiarise the children with the story of *Peter Pan*.

■ Suggest to the children that they use the transformed climbing frame as a pirate ship. Stress that they must remember safety rules while they play. Explain that they should use the ladder to climb on to the ship and leave by going down the slide. For safety reasons, do not include items such as daggers, eye patches or loose clothing such as cloaks.

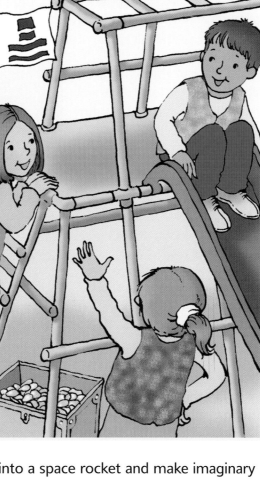

■ As the children play, interact occasionally to extend their imaginary ideas and monitor safe use of the equipment.

■ Use a smaller climbing frame for younger children, and do not introduce the more frightening aspects of piracy.

■ Encourage older children to make up their own stories and negotiate rocks made from climbing cubes as they swim to a 'treasure island'.

## More ideas

■ Transform the climbing frame into a space rocket and make imaginary journeys to the moon.

■ Read some of the *Rosie and Jim* stories by John Cunliffe (Scholastic) and create a narrow boat from various pieces of apparatus.

## Other curriculum areas

MD   Hide ten coins in your room and invite the children to follow clues to search for 'hidden treasure'.

CLL   Act out the story *We're Going on a Bear Hunt* by Michael Rosen (Walker Books) using apparatus to create obstacles.

**Stepping Stone**
Show increasing control in using equipment for climbing, scrambling, sliding and swinging.

**Early Learning Goal**
Use a range of small and large equipment.
■

**Group size**
Four children.
■

**What you need**
The photocopiable sheet 'Ahoy there!' on page 93; climbing frame with ladder and slide attachments; garden cane; white sheeting; black fabric; waistcoats; cardboard box; shiny collage materials such as gold and silver foil; brown paint; copy of *Peter Pan* by J M Barrie (Penguin Books).
■

**Preparation**
Set up the climbing-frame apparatus. Create a flag from white sheeting with black-fabric shapes. Fasten the flag to one corner of the climbing frame with a garden cane. Help the children to make treasure using shiny collage materials, and to paint a cardboard box brown to create a treasure chest.

**Home links**
Give each child a copy of the photocopiable sheet 'Ahoy there!' for them to share with their parents and carers at home.

# Deep in the jungle

Show increasing control in using equipment for climbing, scrambling, sliding and swinging.

**Early Learning Goal**
Use a range of small and large equipment.

**Group size**
Four children.

**What you need**
Climbing frame with slide and ladders attached; safety mats; bench; tunnel; wooden or plastic climbing cubes; carpet tiles; planks of wood; pictures of jungle animals and birds; rope; tissue paper; sticky tape; *Rumble in the Jungle* by Giles Andreae (Orchard Books).

**Preparation**
Set out the apparatus and place carpet tiles at regular intervals so that the children can move easily across them from one piece of equipment to another. Create opportunities for the children to scramble up and down slopes using the planks of wood and slides.

## What to do

▨ Read *Rumble in the Jungle* to the children.

▨ Invite the children to think of ways to make the apparatus that you have arranged look more like a jungle, for example, by draping creepers made from rope and tissue over the tunnel, or by suspending them from the ceiling.

▨ Stick pictures of jungle animals and birds around the area, on walls and screens and in safe places on the apparatus. Avoid accidents by ensuring that parts of the apparatus that the children will be climbing over are kept clear.

▨ Talk about the different animal and bird pictures that the children can see in the jungle as they climb and balance across the apparatus.

▨ Create more gentle slopes for younger children.

▨ Place the bench over some safety mats and pretend that it is a tree that has fallen across a rapidly flowing river. Challenge older children to cross it safely.

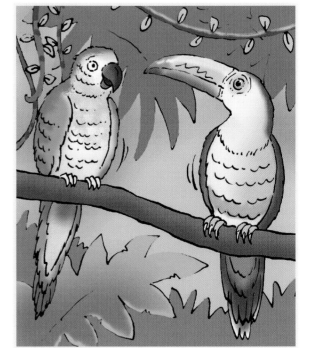

## More ideas

▨ Invite the children to imitate different jungle animals as they move across the apparatus.

▨ Take the children to visit an adventure playground and enjoy negotiating an 'outdoor jungle'.

**Home links**
Encourage parents and carers to take their children to different adventure playgrounds to experience a greater variety of climbing and balancing challenges.

## Other curriculum areas

**KUW** Pretend to be explorers in the jungle carrying a picnic, binoculars, notepad, pencil and camera in a rucksack. Sit down in a clear space to eat the picnic, sketch the animals and birds, and take photographs.

**CD** Use the apparatus as a shipwreck in an undersea world and encourage the children to pretend that they are divers looking for treasure in the wreck.

**Physical development**

# Bowling along

## What to do

▨ Explain how children in the past used to take the metal hoops from wooden barrels and bowl them along the street with a stick. Show the children the pictures.

▨ Invite the children to try to bowl a plastic hoop along with a stick. Encourage them to keep the hoop between the parallel chalk lines and talk about how difficult this is. Is it easier to bowl the hoop along using their hands instead of the stick?

▨ Try bowling rubber or plastic quoits along a flat surface and down slopes.

▨ Push a large plastic barrel across the floor. How easy is this to steer?

▨ Which is easiest to control – the hoop, quoit or barrel?

▨ Let younger children roll just cardboard tubes and rolling-pins along a flat or slightly sloping surface.

▨ Challenge older children by asking them to work in pairs and to bowl a hoop to each other across a clear space.

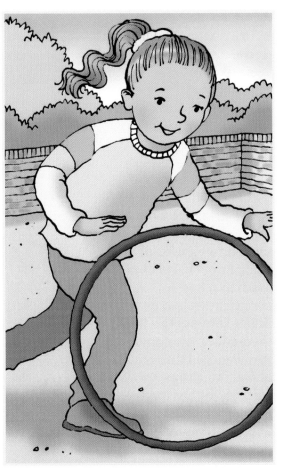

## More ideas

▨ Introduce some simple playground games, for example, 'Hopscotch' and 'Conkers'.

▨ Play 'Cup and ball'. Make a ball from screwed-up paper and a cup from the top half of a plastic drink bottle. Attach the ball to the bottle with string. Use the screw top as a handle to hold the bottle and try to catch the ball in the open end.

---

## Other curriculum areas

**MD** Make some skittles with plastic drink bottles and take turns to roll a ball at them. Count how many are knocked down.

**PSED** Create a role-play fairground. Invent games such as hooking plastic ducks in a water tray using a cane with a ring on the end, or throwing wet sponges at a painting of a clown's face.

---

### Stepping Stone
Use increasing control over an object by touching, pushing, patting, throwing, catching or kicking it.

### Early Learning Goal
Use a range of small and large equipment.
▨

### Group size
Six children.
▨

### What you need
Hard-surfaced outdoor area; hoops; plastic barrels; quoits; sticks or thin branches; thick chalk; pictures of children from the past bowling hoops along with sticks.
▨

### Preparation
Create some parallel tracks on a hard surface outdoors using thick chalk.

### Home links
Invite parents and carers to the role-play fairground and encourage them to take part in the games with their children.

# Bats and balls

## What to do

■ Talk about the resources on the display and encourage the children to tell you how they are used.

■ Suggest to the children that they play with some similar resources.

■ Invite each child to choose a ball from the selection. What does it feel like? Is it easy to hold in one hand, or are two hands needed to pick it up?

■ Explore different ways of handling a ball, for example, pushing or kicking it along the floor, patting it up and down, or throwing it in the air.

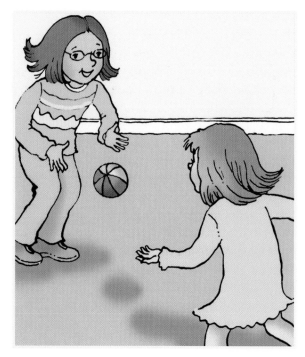

■ Ask the children to work with a partner using one ball between them. Can they throw the ball backwards and forwards? Is it easier to catch a large or a small ball?

■ Allow time for the children to play freely with the balls before introducing the bats.

■ Working with a partner again, invite one child to throw the ball while the other tries to return it with the chosen bat. Try out different combinations of bats and balls.

■ Let younger children use large, light balls that they can catch with two hands, or beanbags that will not roll away from them. Introduce the bats when they can handle the balls with some degree of skill.

■ Encourage older children to try to score goals with a large football.

## More ideas

■ Build towers and roll balls towards them to knock them over.

■ Make an Olympic torch from a cardboard tube and scrunched up paper for the flame. Let the children enjoy running around an open space, passing it from one child to another.

## Other curriculum areas

**MD** Encourage the children to arrange the bats and balls in order of size and to match them by colour.

**PSED** Play a simple version of rounders or cricket with a large bat and a light ball.

**Physical development**

# Roll and catch

## What to do

▨ Invite the children to sit in a circle with their legs apart and their feet touching the child at either side of them.

▨ Explain to the children that you are going to play a game called 'Trap the ball' and that they should try to trap the ball as it comes towards them by closing their legs together. Say that they should not use their hands to catch the ball.

▨ Roll the ball towards one of the children, calling out their name as you do so.

▨ The child who has successfully trapped the ball should then roll it to another child in the circle, calling out the name of the chosen child.

▨ Continue the game until all the children have had a turn. If the children continually choose the same friends, suggest other names, commenting on how these children have been waiting patiently.

▨ Encourage a smaller group of younger children to roll the ball to each other without having to name anyone or aim accurately.

▨ Divide older children into two teams wearing different-coloured bands. Alternate the team members around the circle. Encourage them to roll the ball to a child in the same team. They can score a point when a child in the same team traps the ball, but they lose a point when a child from the opposite team catches it.

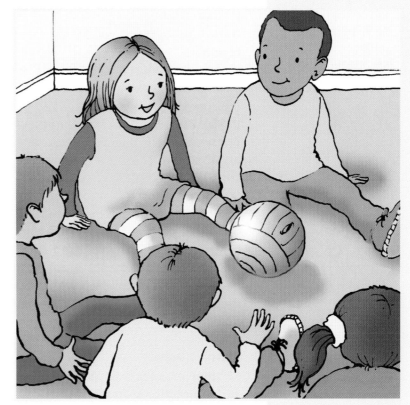

## More ideas

▨ Ask the children to sit in a circle and pass around a beanbag behind their backs.

▨ Pass a quoit from hand to hand around a circle.

**Stepping Stone**
Retrieve, collect and catch objects.

**Early Learning Goal**
Use a range of small and large equipment.
▨
**Group size**
Up to 12 children.
▨
**What you need**
A large ball.

## Other curriculum areas

PSED  Play a team game involving the first child running with a ball and dropping it into a bucket, then sitting beside it. The next child in the team should then do the same, until all the players have had a turn.

MD  Pretend to be potato pickers running around a 'field' of beanbag 'potatoes', picking them up and putting them in a bucket. Challenge the children to pick up as many as possible in a given time.

Home links
Hold a simple sports day. Invite parents and carers to come to watch and encourage them to participate in fun races.

*Physical development*

# Beanbag race

## What to do
▨ Mix up the coloured beanbags and ask the children to sort them into a red pile and a yellow pile.
▨ Put the two storage containers at the end of a clear space.
▨ Invite the children to each choose a coloured band and put it on.
▨ Spread the red beanbags evenly between the children and the red storage container.
▨ Repeat with the yellow beanbags.
▨ Ask the children to sit in a row next to the beanbags that match the colour of the bands that they are wearing.

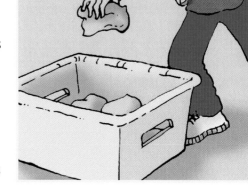

▨ Invite the first child in each row to pick up a beanbag, run, drop the beanbag into the corresponding container and return to the back of the line. Ask the next child to do the same, until all the children have picked up and dropped a beanbag.
▨ With younger children, do not have teams; simply distribute the beanbags randomly around the floor with the two containers in the centre and invite the children to pick up the beanbags one by one and return them to the appropriate containers.
▨ Provide older children with a bucket to put the beanbag in and ask them to pass the bucket to the next child, until all of the beanbags are in a bucket.

## More ideas
▨ Steer a buggy or pram in and out of a row of cones to collect a doll and bring it back again.
▨ Blow bubbles and ask the children to try to burst them by clapping their hands.

## Other curriculum areas
| CD | Print with sponge balls by rolling them across paper or by pressing them down, then lifting them up. |
| KUW | Explore the behaviour of different balls, including sponge and plastic airflow balls, in a water tray. |

**Physical development**

This chapter suggests ideas to enable the children to handle a variety of tools, objects and construction and malleable materials, such as marbles, clay, woodwork tools and kitchen utensils, safely and with increasing control.

# Marble fun

Goals for the
Foundation
Stage

**Stepping Stone**
Engage in activities requiring hand–eye co-ordination.

**Early Learning Goal**
Handle tools, objects, construction and malleable materials safely and with increasing control.

**Group size**
Four children.

**What you need**
Four shallow plastic trays; different-coloured thick paints; four marbles; paper; scissors; small plastic dishes; aprons.

## What to do
■ Cut the paper so that it fits into the trays.
■ Put a small amount of different-coloured paint into each small dish and arrange the dishes in a row in the centre of the table.
■ Place a marble into each dish of paint.
■ Ask the children to put on the aprons, then give each child a tray and ensure that a good supply of paper is readily accessible for them to use.
■ Demonstrate to the children how to lift the marble out of the dish and drop it on to the paper in the tray.
■ Allow plenty of time for the children to explore what happens when they move the tray around with the marble inside.
■ Let younger children dip sponge balls into the paint and encourage them to try rolling or dabbing them across a sheet of paper.
■ Challenge older children by asking them to make their marbles go round and round in their trays. Bear in mind the learning objective of controlling the tray to make the marble move in the desired direction as you ask the questions.

## More ideas
■ Create string patterns by dipping a piece of string into some thick paint and arranging it on half of a piece of paper with the end protruding from one corner. Fold the other half of the paper on top, press down hard with one hand and pull the string out with the other. Open the paper out to reveal the pattern.
■ Dip a paintbrush into some runny paint and create splash-paint patterns by holding the paintbrush over a piece of paper with one hand and flicking it with the other.

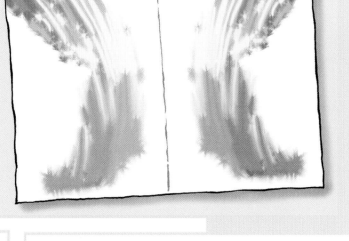

## Other curriculum areas
**MD** Roll marbles down slopes and try to get them through arches cut in small cardboard boxes, numbered 1 to 5.

**PSED** Take turns to pick up as many marbles as possible with a spoon before a sand-timer runs out.

**Home links**
Give each child a sheet to take home explaining to parents and carers how to set up the activity using ordinary household resources. Explain the learning objective for the activity and suggest appropriate questions for parents and carers to ask their children to promote this objective.

# Into pairs

### Early Learning Goal
Handle tools, objects, construction and malleable materials safely and with increasing control.

### Group size
Four children.

### What you need
The photocopiable sheet 'Odd one out' on page 94; several pairs of socks of different sizes and colours, plain as well as with a variety of patterns; washing line; pegs; peg basket; washing basket.

### Preparation
Mix up the socks and put them in the washing basket. Suspend the washing line so that the children can easily reach it. Make sure that it is not too low for safety reasons.

### Home links
Ask parents and carers to encourage their children to pair socks and to hang out washing at home.

## What to do
■ Sit in a circle around the washing basket and ask the children to tell you what sort of items they think you have been washing.
■ Explain that the socks have become mixed up in the wash and that you would like the children to help you to sort them into pairs again.
■ Invite the children to take turns to pull out a pair of matching socks, then to go to the washing line and hang them up, still in matching pairs.
■ Continue to pick out pairs of socks and hang them up, until they all have been sorted.

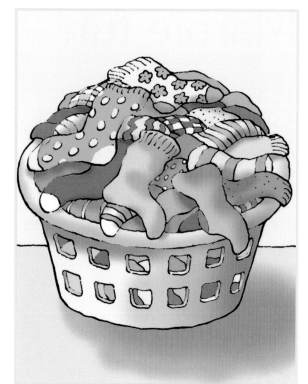

■ Give each child a copy of the photocopiable sheet. Ask them to put a large cross through the odd sock in each line and to colour in the matching two.
■ Give younger children fewer and more definite choices, for example, a pair of large brightly patterned socks and a pair of tiny white babies' socks. Also make sure that the pegs are easy enough for their small fingers to manipulate.
■ Provide older children with a selection of pegs, such as spring-clip pegs, plastic push-on pegs and wooden 'dolly' pegs.

## More ideas
■ Wash the dolls' clothes from the home area and hang them out to dry.
■ Create patterns with pegs and pegboards of varying sizes, and complete puzzles with peg inserts.

## Other curriculum areas
MD Sort a basket of washing, for example, babies' clothes and children's clothes, or sort and match a basket of clothes by colour. Hang up the clothes in separate groups.

PSED Encourage the children's concentration skills by asking them to try to pick up very small items, for example, rice grains, with a pair of tweezers.

**Physical development**

# Painted fences

## What to do

■ Look at the pictures and talk to the children about the work of painters. Have they ever seen a painter working outside, painting doors, windows or fences? What do painters wear? Talk about the need to protect clothes and hair with overalls, aprons and hats.

■ Suggest to the children that they pretend to be painters, painting the outside of the building or the fences. Invite them to put on the aprons and hats.

■ Show the children the selection of paintbrushes. Which paintbrushes do the children think would be most suitable to paint a fence? Could they use a thin paintbrush that they use at your setting? Would it cover the surface easily?

■ Ask each child to choose a paintbrush to take outside. Find a flat surface to paint and give each child a bucket of water.

■ Let the children 'paint' freely, exchanging brushes and painting different surfaces.

■ Give younger children smaller buckets of water and suitable brushes (not too large).

■ Encourage older children to create wavy and straight-line patterns with their paintbrushes, or to try to write some of the letters in their names.

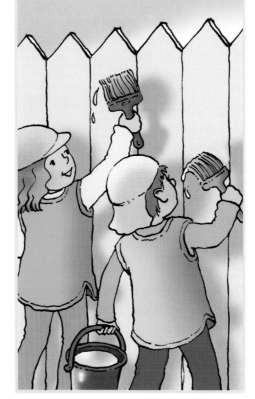

## More ideas

■ Invite the children to paint wavy and straight-line patterns on to paper using paintbrushes from your setting of various thicknesses.

■ Suggest that the children paint pictures and patterns using unusual paintbrushes, such as washing-up brushes, toothbrushes and bottle brushes. Do not use old brushes, to prevent the possibility of infection.

---

### Other curriculum areas

CLL  Invite the children to use a stick to write the letters of their names in sand, or in thick paint spread across a sheet of paper

KUW  Investigate how water evaporates in the sun and wind by inviting the children to 'paint' areas of a fence in the shade and in direct sunlight. Which area is the fastest to dry?

---

**Stepping Stone**
Use one-handed tools and equipment.

**Early Learning Goal**
Handle tools, objects, construction and malleable materials safely and with increasing control.
■
**Group size**
Six children.
■
**What you need**
Pictures of people painting houses; household paintbrushes of different sizes; paintbrushes from your setting; buckets; water; aprons; caps or sun-hats.

**Home links**
Suggest to parents and carers that they encourage their children to use tools and equipment around the house, under their supervision, when the opportunity arises.

---

**Physical development**

# Tiny and giant workers

**Stepping Stone**
Use one-handed tools and equipment.

**Early Learning Goal**
Handle tools, objects, construction and malleable materials safely and with increasing control.

**Group size**
Four children.

**What you need**
Small tools and utensils to pick up tiny objects, such as tweezers, mustard spoons and sugar tongs; large tools and utensils to pick up larger objects, such as barbecue tongs, tablespoons and scoops; tiny objects, such as peas, sunflower seeds, rice grains and buttons; larger objects, such as table-tennis balls, plastic bricks and small plastic bears; large and small plastic bowls; two tables.

**Preparation**
Put the tiny objects into separate small bowls in the centre of a table with the small tools, utensils and empty bowls alongside them. Do the same with the larger objects, tools, utensils and bowls on another table.

## What to do
■ Show the children the resources on each table. What do they notice about the differences in size of the items?
■ Invite two children to work at each table and encourage them to try to lift up the objects with the various tools and utensils and transfer them into empty bowls.
■ Suggest to the children that they change places and work at the other table.
■ Talk about which items were easiest to pick up and which were the most difficult. What do they think would happen if they tried to pick up a tiny object with a large utensil?
■ Do not give young children very small items to pick up, for safety reasons. Use larger resources only at first to develop their confidence.
■ Challenge older children to count how many small objects they can pick up in a given time.

## More ideas
■ Transfer objects to a bucket balance using different utensils, such as scoops and spoons, and try to make both buckets weigh the same.
■ Sew simple hand puppets using an open-weave fabric, thick wool and blunt needles.

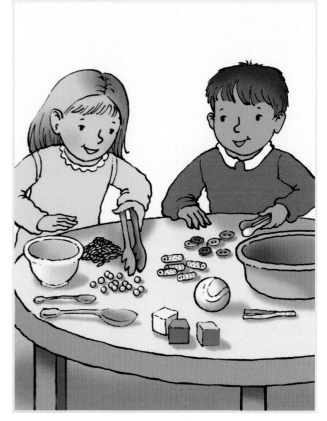

**Home links**
Encourage parents and carers to let their children weigh and measure ingredients during baking sessions, using different scoops and spoons of varying sizes.

## Other curriculum areas
CD Encourage the children to work with clay using a variety of tools and objects to create different surface patterns.
PSED Invite the children to use chopsticks when sampling Chinese food during a related festival. Check for any food allergies and dietary requirements.

# Parking places

## What to do

■ Ask the children to each choose a small car from the selection. Talk about cars that the children have ridden in. Do their parents or carers have a car, or do they know anyone else who has one? Where do the owners of the cars put them to keep them safe and dry?

■ Talk about car garages. Do the children have a garage? Suggest that they use the construction equipment available to make garages for their chosen cars.

■ Interact with the children as they work. Suggest ways in which they can ensure that the garage is a suitable size, and help them to construct the roof.

■ Invite the children to place the cars inside the garages, then take them out again and talk about how to ensure that each car returns to the same garage.

■ Suggest to the children that they create matching labels for their cars and garages and attach them with sticky tape.

■ Play games with a road mat, pushing the cars around it and returning them to the correct garages at the end of the journey.

■ Let younger children each make a simple mark, such as a happy face, on each label to identify their car and garage.

■ Encourage older children to write their names on the labels.

## More ideas

■ Invite the children to create shelters for small-world animals using different types of construction equipment.

■ Draw roads and rail tracks on to a large sheet of card. Use this as a basis for imaginary play with small-world characters and equipment.

## Other curriculum areas

MD  Make number labels for the cars and garages and match them together.

CLL  Make up stories about imaginary journeys in the cars using other small-world props such as animals and people.

### Stepping Stone
Demonstrate increasing skill and control in the use of mark-making implements, blocks, construction sets and 'small world' activities.

### Early Learning Goal
Handle tools, objects, construction and malleable materials safely and with increasing control.

■

### Group size
Four children.

■

### What you need
Large container of plastic construction equipment; selection of small cars; white card; sticky tape; scissors; felt-tipped pens.

■

### Preparation
Cut the white card into rectangles, small enough to attach to the cars.

### Home links
Explain the learning objective of this activity to parents and carers and suggest that they play with a variety of construction equipment with their children at home.

**Physical development**

# Down on the farm

**Stepping Stone**
Demonstrate increasing skill and control in the use of mark-making implements, blocks, construction sets and 'small world' activities.

**Early Learning Goal**
Handle tools, objects, construction and malleable materials safely and with increasing control.

**Group size**
Four children.

**What you need**
Small-world farm animals and people; fences from a farm set; plastic construction equipment; floor mat with a countryside scene of fields, farm tracks and roads; paper; sticky tape.

**Home links**
Suggest to parents and carers that they take their children to visit a farm park to see all the different animals.

## What to do
■ Talk about the children's experiences of farms. Invite them to name the small-world farm animals and sort them into groups.
■ Discuss how the animals are separated on a farm. What prevents them from escaping from the fields? Where do they go when it is cold and wet?
■ Link some fencing around the edge of a field on the floor mat. Decide together which type of animal will live in the field and invite the children to put those animals into it.
■ Continue creating fields until all the groups of farm animals are in separate enclosures.
■ Make some barns using construction equipment, for the animals to shelter in.
■ Have fewer animals for younger children to sort, and help them to link the fences.
■ Invite older children to create labels for the enclosures by drawing the animals and writing captions alongside. Attach the labels with sticky tape and encourage the children to put the farm animals into the correct enclosures.

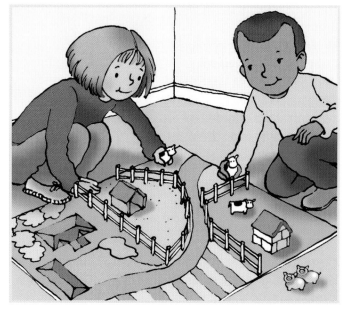

## More ideas
■ Use building blocks to create caves for model dinosaurs.
■ Make road signs from lollipop sticks with small pieces of card glued to the top. Copy pictures or words from familiar road signs and stand the finished signs in clay. Position them on a small-world road mat.

## Other curriculum areas
CLL  Make name tiles by rolling out flat squares of clay. Ask the children to write their names or initials by pressing a clay tool on to the surface to create an impression. Bake the tiles until hard.
MD  Attach the numbers 1 to 10 to a line of blocks, then build a tower in numerical order. See how many blocks can be stacked by looking at the number on the top block just before the tower falls.

**Physical development**

# Super soup

## What to do

■ Talk about any soups that the children enjoy and suggest that they make some soup for their friends.

■ Ask them to wash their hands and put on aprons.

■ Discuss each utensil in turn and demonstrate how it is used, for example, scrub clean a small piece of carrot and grate it, or peel part of a potato.

■ Name each vegetable and put it in the centre of the table, along with the utensils. Give each child a chopping board and invite them to prepare the vegetables and put them into the saucepan. Supervise them carefully and emphasise the safe handling of tools, especially the grater, knife and peeler.

■ Invite a child to crumble a stock cube into a jug of warm water and pour it into the saucepan.

■ Cover the vegetables and boil them, away from the children, until they are cooked.

■ Allow the soup to cool before serving.

■ Let younger children scrub the vegetables for older children and adults to cut up.

■ Encourage older children to try as many different tools and utensils as possible, under supervision, for example, flat and round graters.

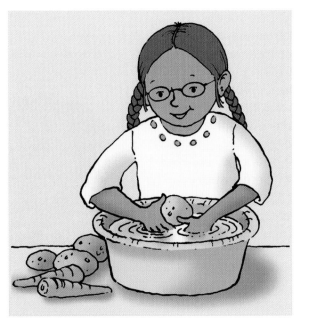

## More ideas

■ Make comparisons between using a hand whisk and a hand-held electric mixer to whisk some cream.

■ Try unusual combinations of flavours such as carrot and orange soup. Chop up some carrots and mix them with the juice and zest of an orange. Add extra water to cover, and simmer for 20 minutes. Season with nutmeg and lemon juice, then liquidise.

## Other curriculum areas

KUW  Show the children how to liquidise soup or heat it in a microwave oven.

CLL  Make laminated pictorial recipe cards for different types of soup.

## Home links
Send home a pictorial sheet of soup recipes for parents and carers to try with their children at home.

### Stepping Stone
Understand that equipment and tools have to be used safely.

### Early Learning Goal
Handle tools, objects, construction and malleable materials safely and with increasing control.

■

### Group size
Four children.

■

### What you need
Cooker; fresh vegetables such as a potato, carrot, turnip, cabbage and onion; vegetable-stock cube; jug; warm water; large saucepan; four chopping boards; four kitchen knives (not too sharp); small scrubbing brushes; cheese grater; potato peeler; well-illustrated recipe book; aprons.

■

### Preparation
Cut large vegetables into smaller pieces beforehand for easier handling. Check for any food allergies and dietary requirements.

# Working with wood

Understand that equipment and tools have to be used safely.

## Early Learning Goal
Handle tools, objects, construction and malleable materials safely and with increasing control.

## Group size
Six children to demonstrate how to use the equipment; two children to work at the woodwork bench.

## What you need
Woodwork bench; two clamp-on vices; two small hammers; nails with flat heads; two small tenon saws; two bradawls; sandpaper blocks; pliers; wood offcuts; box for wood; woodwork aprons.

## Preparation
Position the woodwork bench away from quiet activities and screened off if possible, for safety. Display the tools on a table and store the wood offcuts in a box underneath. Hang the aprons on the screen.

## What to do
■ Explain to the children about the need for simple rules in the woodwork area, for example, always wearing aprons and only having one child working at each vice.
■ Demonstrate to the children how to use the tools safely and return them to their designated places after use.
■ Invite two children to choose a piece of wood from the container and suggest that the others return later when there is space at the bench. Show the children how to clamp the wood into a vice and allow time for them to explore the tools that are available.
■ Let younger children simply sand wood offcuts to make them smooth. Suggest that they take them away to paint or glue small items on to them, for example, milk-bottle tops, buttons and seeds.
■ Once older children are working confidently, extend their skills by introducing additional tools such as a manual hand drill, flat plane and screwdriver. Ensure that they handle the tools correctly at all times.

## More ideas
■ Roll a small branch across a piece of play dough to make unusual prints.
■ Create imaginary creatures from branches, using recyclable materials such as buttons, fabric scraps and twigs to create features and limbs.

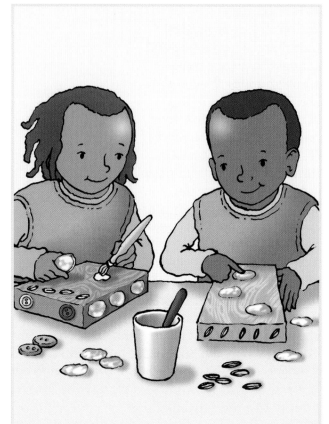

## Home links
Ask parents and carers to take their children on a hunt for wooden objects around their home.

## Other curriculum areas
KUW Examine the features of logs, such as the annual rings and outer bark, with a magnifying glass, then make observational drawings.

MD Sort a box of pieces of wood according to length, shape, weight or texture.

# Fun with dough

## What to do

■ Tell the children that you are going to make some play dough and that you would like them to help you. Invite them to put on aprons, then show them the pictorial recipe card. Look at it and gather together the appropriate ingredients and utensils.

■ Ask individual children to weigh out 200g of plain flour and 100g of salt, and to measure out two teaspoons of cream of tartar and one tablespoon of cooking oil. Put all the ingredients into the saucepan.

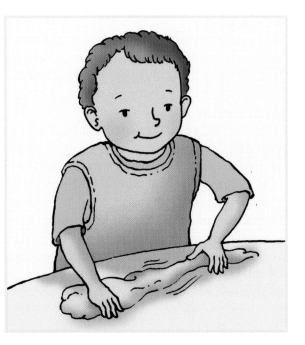

■ Invite a child to measure 300ml of water in a jug and to add a few drops of food colouring to it before pouring it gently into the pan.

■ Let the children take turns to stir the mixture.

■ Heat the mixture slowly away from the children, until it forms a stiff ball. Tip it on to a pastry board and leave it to cool.

■ Divide the play dough equally among the children and let them play with it without tools. Encourage them to try patting, stroking, poking, squeezing, pinching and twisting it.

■ With younger children, omit making the dough and concentrate on spending time playing freely with a ready-made batch, using different finger and hand movements.

■ Encourage older children to mix together self-raising flour and water to make their own 'stretchy' dough.

## More ideas

■ Add different textures and scents to the cold dough mixture, for example, rolled oats and lemon essence.

■ Introduce unusual tools to use with the play dough, such as a pastry wheel, garlic press and potato masher.

## Other curriculum areas

MD  Create dough snakes of different lengths and introduce appropriate language, such as 'longest', 'shorter' and 'same as'.

CLL  Form dough snakes into the initial letters of the children's names and bake them to create badges.

## Stepping Stone
Explore malleable materials by patting, stroking, poking, squeezing, pinching and twisting them.

## Early Learning Goal
Handle tools, objects, construction and malleable materials safely and with increasing control.

■

## Group size
Four children.

■

## What you need
Cooker; plain flour; salt; cream of tartar; cooking oil; water; different-coloured food colourings; scales; teaspoon; tablespoon; bowls; shallow dish; jug; large saucepan; sieve; four pastry boards; aprons.

■

## Preparation
Create a pictorial recipe card that the children can refer to as they make their play dough.

## Home links
Send home a copy of the photocopiable sheet 'Play-dough recipe' on page 95, so that parents and carers can make it with their children at home.

# Diva lamps

## Stepping Stone
Manipulate materials to achieve a planned effect.

## Early Learning Goal
Handle tools, objects, construction and malleable materials safely and with increasing control.

## Group size
Six children.

## What you need
Pictures about the festival of Divali showing diva lamps; clay; clay tools; paint; PVA glue; tea lights.

## What to do
■ Explain the importance of lights during the festival of Divali, which is celebrated in October or November each year by Sikhs and Hindus, and how Divali means 'a row (or cluster) of lights'.
■ Suggest to the children that they make their own diva lamps to display on the window sills.
■ Invite each child to form a ball of clay by rolling it around in the palms of their hands.
■ Explain to the children how to put the ball into the palm of one hand and to press into the centre with the thumb from the other hand until they form a bowl shape.
■ Put the bowl on the table, press it down to form a flat base and widen it further by pressing around the side. Make sure that the centre of the bowl is big enough to accommodate a tea light. Create a lip on the side of the bowl.
■ Allow the finished bowl, or diva lamp, to dry a little before etching patterns on the side with clay tools.
■ Invite the children to paint their lamps and, once dry, cover them with a layer of PVA glue to give a varnished appearance.
■ Place a tea light in the centre of each bowl.
■ Display the lamps as part of a Divali table display.

■ Let younger children simply explore how they can manipulate a lump of clay rather than concentrate on an end product.
■ Encourage older children to extend their skills by making coiled pots.

## More ideas
■ Make clay pots at other times of the year, for example, to house bulbs or seeds in spring, or for Christmas table decorations.
■ Light the diva lamps on a dull afternoon, in a safe place away from the children's reach. Tell stories to the children by lamplight.

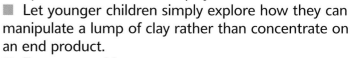

## Home links
Send home a copy of the photocopiable sheet 'The Divali story' on page 96, together with the children's diva lamps. Ask parents and carers to read the story to their children by candlelight.

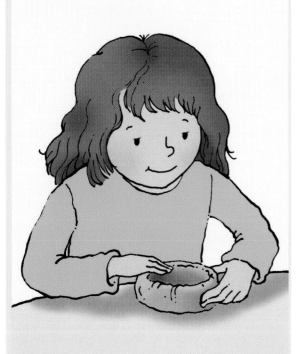

## Other curriculum areas
KUW — Create diva lamps and bowls from papier mâché.
CD — Make a thick flour paste and spread it on a table. Create patterns on the surface with fingers and card combs.

# Snowy days

## What to do
■ Take the children outside on a snowy day and talk about how things look when they are covered in a blanket of snow. If there is enough snow, build different snow characters together. Alternatively, talk about the children's experiences of snowy days as part of topics on 'Winter', 'Seasons' or 'Weather'.

■ Give each child a sheet of black paper and encourage them to create a snowman, or character of their choice, on the paper using the resources available. They might like to paint a snow cat or rabbit, or cut something out of white paper to glue on to the black paper.

■ Suggest to the children that they create some snow by cutting sheets of white paper into tiny pieces. Cover the whole of the black paper and the children's snow characters with glue so that they can sprinkle their 'snow' all over the paper to create a snowstorm effect.

■ Let younger children tear the white paper rather than cut it.

■ Show older children how to curl strips of white paper and glue them to black paper to form three-dimensional pictures, for example, of a sheep in the snow.

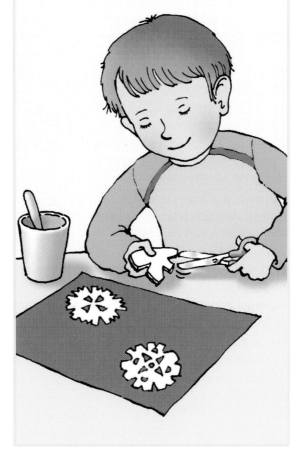

## More ideas
■ Organise similar activities with different-coloured papers at various times of the year to create seasonal pictures, such as autumn leaves or spring blossom falling from trees.

■ Make paper snowflakes by folding paper circles in half and then into thirds. Cut small pieces out of the sides, and then open out the circles.

## Other curriculum areas
CD Create a stained-glass window effect by attaching different-coloured tissue paper to a black-paper frame and putting it in front of a window.

PSED Make paper chains and streamers to decorate rooms at festival times.

**Home links**
Encourage parents and carers to purchase small scissors for their children and to help them to practise their cutting skills at home by cutting out pictures from old catalogues.

**Physical development**

# I can manage!

**Stepping Stone**
Show understanding
of how to transport
and store equipment
safely.

### Early Learning Goal
Handle tools,
objects, construction
and malleable
materials safely and
with increasing
control.

### Group size
Four children.

### What you need
Two painting easels;
paint; paint pots;
paintbrushes; paper;
pencils; string;
aprons; paint drying
rack; hand-washing
facilities.

### Preparation
Fasten a piece of
string to each pencil
and attach the
pencils to the
painting easels.

### Home links
Encourage parents
and carers to involve
their children in
transporting things
at home, such as
putting the shopping
away.

## What to do
■ Talk to the children about painting a picture. What do they do first? What is the last thing that they do?

■ Suggest to the children that they paint a picture so that everyone knows exactly what to do from beginning to end.

■ Start by putting on aprons. Can the children reach an apron, put it on and fasten it? If necessary, adapt your storage of aprons and fastenings so that the children can put on the aprons independently.

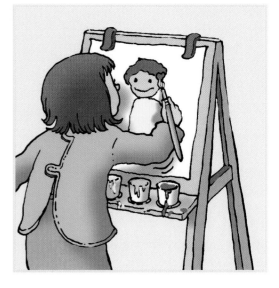

■ Ask the children to each get a piece of paper. Do they know where to find a piece of paper and how to fasten it to an easel? Again, adapt storage and fastening methods, if necessary.

■ When the children paint a picture, do they return the paintbrushes to the correct pots? If necessary, explain how to do this.

■ Once the pictures are finished, encourage the children to write their names or indicate that it is their picture with an identity mark, using the pencil attached to the easel.

■ Invite the children to take their paintings from the easel to the drying rack. Can they reach all equipment easily?

■ Ask the children to wash their hands and emphasise the need to wash them thoroughly.

■ Make sure that the easels are low enough for younger children to reach the top. Help them to attach the paper to the easel and to wash their hands if necessary.

■ Invite older children to assist with mixing the paints and setting up supplies of paper for the paint easels.

## More ideas
■ Encourage the children follow to simple safety rules when helping to transport the outdoor equipment.

■ Label storage containers with pictures and words so that the children can put things away easily.

## Other curriculum areas
KUW Ask the children to help you make signs for each play area in your setting, using a computer, printer and laminator.

PSED Leave a 'helper's choice' table clear at the start of each session and ask the children who are 'daily helpers' to set up their own choice of activity on it.

# Physical development (1)

Name _____

| Goals | Assessment | Date |
|---|---|---|
| **Movement** | | |
| Move with confidence, imagination and in safety. | | |
| Move with control and co-ordination. | | |
| Travel around, under, over and through balancing and climbing equipment. | | |
| **Sense of space** | | |
| Show awareness of space, of themselves and of others. | | |

# Physical development (2)

Name _____

| Goals | Assessment | Date |
|---|---|---|
| **Health and bodily awareness** | | |
| Recognise the importance of keeping healthy and those things which contribute to this. | | |
| Recognise the changes that happen to their bodies when they are active. | | |
| **Using equipment** | | |
| Use a range of small and large equipment. | | |
| **Using tools and materials** | | |
| Handle tools, objects, construction and malleable materials safely and with increasing control. | | |

# Weather rhymes

### I Hear Thunder, I Hear Thunder
I hear thunder, I hear thunder;
Hark, don't you, Hark, don't you?
Pitter-patter raindrops,
Pitter-patter raindrops,
I'm wet through,
SO ARE YOU!

Traditional

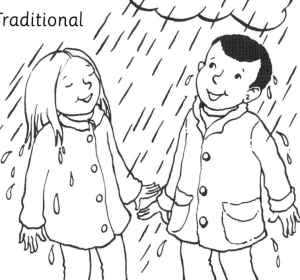

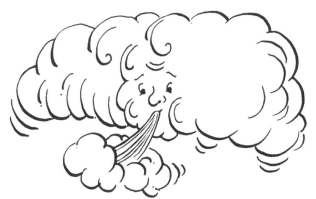

### The North Wind Doth Blow
The North Wind doth blow
And we shall have snow,
And what will the robin do then,
Poor thing?
He'll sleep in the barn,
To keep himself warm,
And hide his head under his wing,
Poor thing!

Traditional

### Here We Go Round the Mulberry Bush
Here we go round the Mulberry Bush,
The Mulberry Mush, the Mulberry Bush;
Here we go round the Mulberry Bush,
On a cold and frosty morning.

We stamp our feet to keep them warm,
Stamp our feet to keep them warm;
We stamp our feet to keep them warm,
On a cold and frosty morning.

Traditional

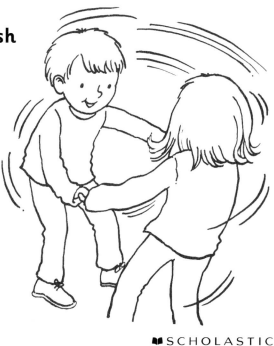

**Physical development**

**Photocopiable**

■SCHOLASTIC

# Little learners

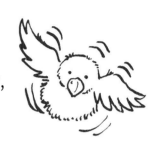

*Tune: 'Five Little Speckled Frogs'*

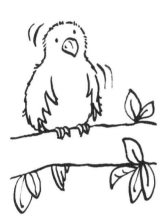
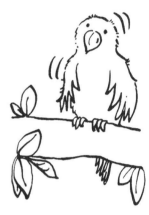

Five little baby crows, sat in a little row,
Wishing that they knew how to fly,
Caw, caw.
One jumped down to the ground,
Where he/she flapped round and round,
Then he/she took off into the sky,
Caw, caw.

Four little baby crows... *(and so on)*

Three little baby crows... *(and so on)*

Two little baby crows... *(and so on)*

One little baby crow... *(and so on)*

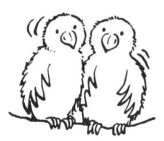
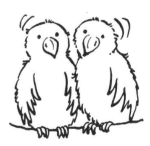

No little baby crows, sat in a little row,
Wishing that they knew how to fly,
Caw, caw.
They all flew round and round,
High up above the ground,
Happy that they knew how to fly,
Caw, caw.

Jean Evans

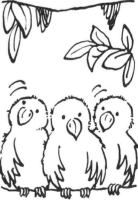

Find the way home

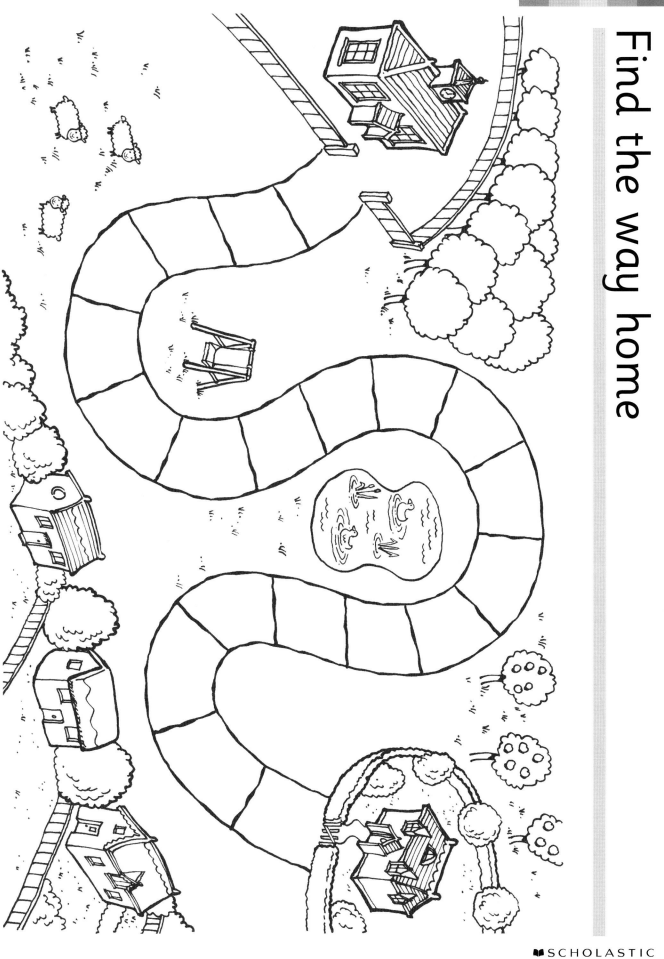

Photocopiable

◢SCHOLASTIC

# What a journey!

The Green family were very excited because they were moving to their new house across the wide river, through the deep tunnel and over the tall hill. Off they went, following the big removal van rumbling down the road. Inside the old house everything was quiet… except for a low rumbling sound. What could it be? In the bathroom, at the bottom of the warm airing cupboard, slept Isla the cat, snoring peacefully. The family had forgotten to take her in their hurry!

Isla woke up, stretched herself lazily and padded downstairs to search for food. Where was everyone? She waved her tail and twitched her whiskers. Her food and water bowls were empty. She pushed through her cat flap in the kitchen door and went outside.

She sniffed the air.

'The family went this way,' she miaowed, stalking down the road until she came to a wide river. *(safety mats)*

'I hate swimming,' she hissed. 'How can I cross the water?'

Soon she spotted some smooth stones. *(hoops on mats)*

She jumped easily from one stone to the next until she reached the dry bank at the other side of the river.

She sniffed the air.

'The family went this way,' she miaowed, stalking down the road until she came to a deep tunnel.

'I don't like dark places,' she hissed. 'How can I get through this tunnel?' She looked through and found that she could see the other side. Happily she crawled right through the tunnel and out again.

She sniffed the air.

'The family went this way,' she miaowed, stalking down the road until she came to a tall hill.

*(wooden climbing steps)*

'I don't like climbing hills,' she hissed. 'How can I get to the other side?'

Luckily she spotted some steps in the hillside and easily climbed up them. She sniffed the air.

'The family went this way,' she miaowed, stalking down the road until she came to a winding path.

She purred to herself, 'I can easily run along this path,' and so she did. Suddenly she heard her name being called, 'Isla, Isla, where are you?'

In the distance she could see a house with all of her family standing outside.

'Isla, Isla, you are home!' they said, patting and stroking her all at once.

'This doesn't look like my home,' thought Isla, 'but if my family are here then I'm happy'.

Jean Evans

# Where is my burrow?

Hoppity the rabbit was enjoying himself. Hoppity, hop, hoppity hop, he went, down from his burrow in the green, green meadow and into the deep, dark woods.

'I am hungry,' he said. 'Where is my burrow in the green, green meadow?'

Hoppity looked around. No green, green meadow, only a hole in the ground in front of him.

Rustle, creak... from down in the hole shuffled a sleepy mole.

'Hello, who are you?' asked Hoppity. 'I'm hungry and I can't find my burrow in the green, green meadow.'

'I'm a sleepy mole in my tunnel. I'm sorry I can't help you. Why not ask the frog in the pond? He knows lots of things.'

The mole shuffled back into the dark tunnel... rustle, creak... and disappeared.

Hoppity looked around. No green, green meadow. He hopped along until he came to a round pond.

Splish, splosh, out of the deep water jumped a shiny speckled frog.

'Hello, who are you?' asked Hoppity. 'I'm hungry and I can't find my burrow in the green, green meadow.'

'I'm a shiny frog in my pond. I'm sorry I can't help you. Why not ask the hedgehog in the leaves? He knows lots of things.'

The frog jumped across the lily pads... one, two, three and four... and disappeared.

Hoppity looked around. No green, green meadow. He hopped along until he came to a pile of leaves.

Crunch, scrunch... out of the leaves rolled a prickly, twitchy hedgehog.

'Hello, who are you?' asked Hoppity. 'I'm hungry and I can't find my burrow in the green, green meadow.'

'I'm a prickly hedgehog in my pile of leaves. I'm sorry I can't help you. Why not go along the path? It seems lighter that way.'

The hedgehog rolled over and over in the leaves and disappeared.

Hoppity looked around. No green, green meadow, but a winding path leading back into the light. He hopped along and there was the green, green meadow, and his mum hopping in front of their burrow waiting for him to come home for his dinner!

Jean Evans

# Funny faces

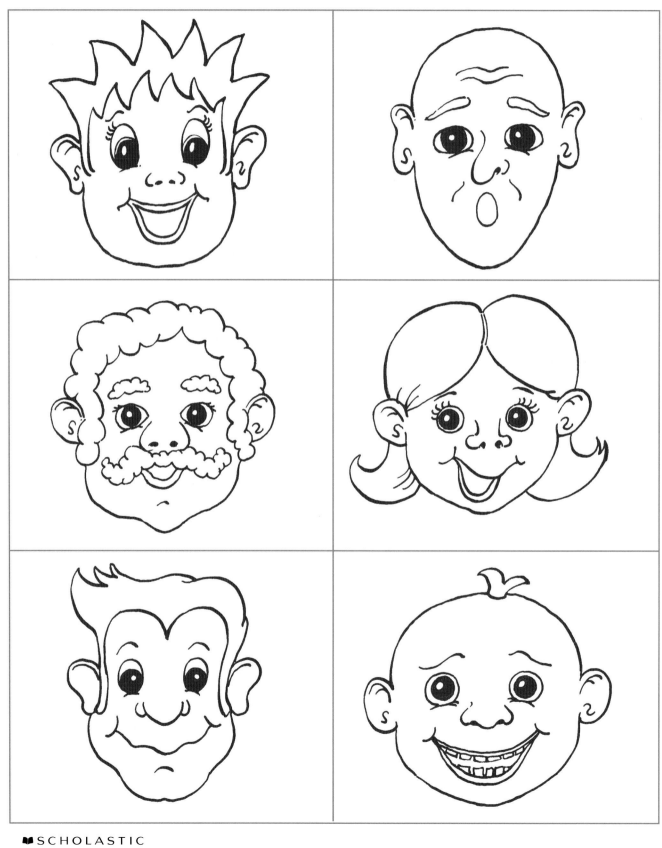

**Photocopiable**

**Physical development**

# Our rules

The following list is only a guide to setting out rules. It is suggested that you add extra points related to your setting and remove any that you feel are inappropriate.

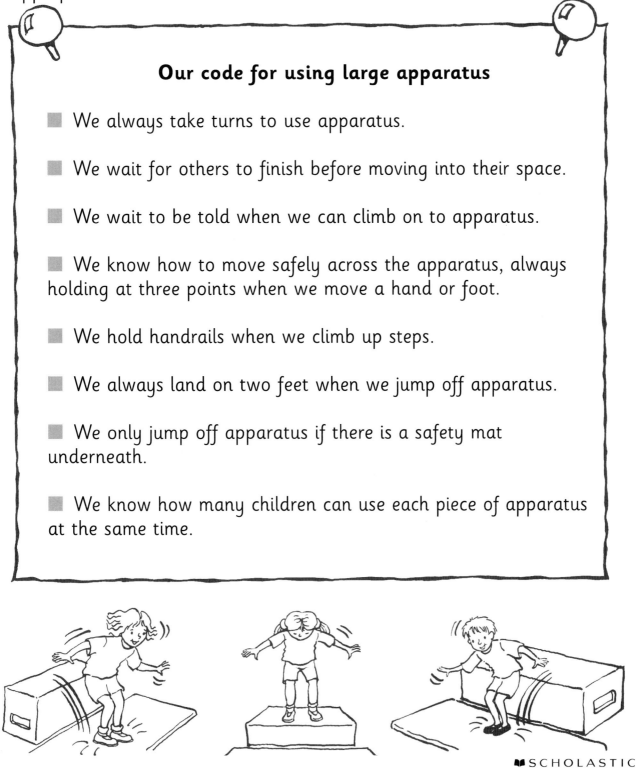

## Our code for using large apparatus

- We always take turns to use apparatus.

- We wait for others to finish before moving into their space.

- We wait to be told when we can climb on to apparatus.

- We know how to move safely across the apparatus, always holding at three points when we move a hand or foot.

- We hold handrails when we climb up steps.

- We always land on two feet when we jump off apparatus.

- We only jump off apparatus if there is a safety mat underneath.

- We know how many children can use each piece of apparatus at the same time.

**SCHOLASTIC**

# Regular routines

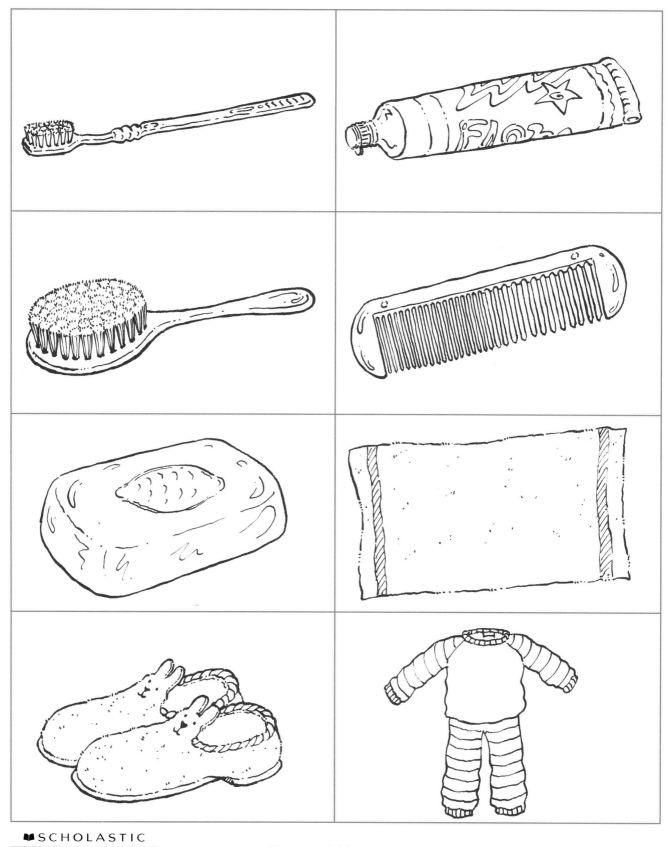

**Photocopiable**

**Physical development**

Dressed for the weather

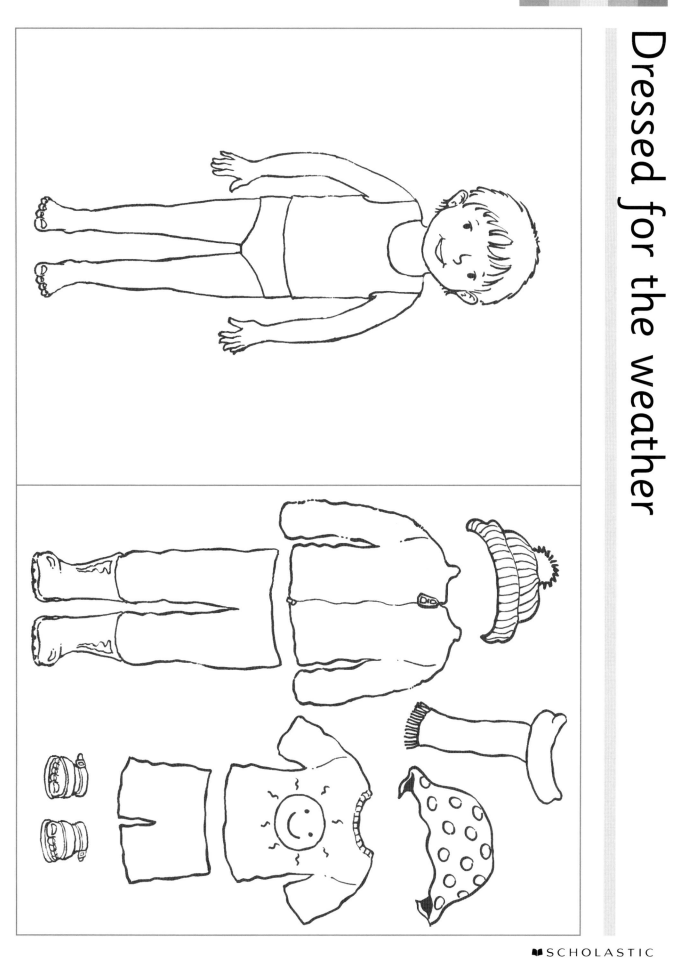

Photocopiable

SCHOLASTIC

89

# Muffin pizzas

The children have been learning about keeping healthy and the things that contribute to this, such as a healthy diet. Why not try making these simple pizzas at home using muffins instead of pizza dough? Remember to involve your child as much as possible at every stage.

## You will need

Muffins (one muffin makes two small pizzas); tomato purée; toppings of your own choice, such as cheese, small tomatoes, sweetcorn, green, yellow and red peppers, cooked sausages or sliced ham and mushrooms; cheese grater; chopping board; knife (not too sharp); baking tray; small bowl; boiling water (adult use); grill (adult use). For vegetarian pizzas, simply omit the meat.

### Things to talk about with your child

■ How pizzas are good to eat because they are made of a lot of healthy foods.
■ The names of all the ingredients.
■ The importance of eating fresh vegetables.
■ How cheese helps bones and teeth to grow strong.
■ How bread gives us energy.

## What to do

■ Prepare the tomatoes beforehand by plunging them in a bowl of boiling water until the skins split before peeling them. Do this away from your child for safety reasons.

■ Give your child a muffin and invite him/her to cut the muffin in half, then make a sauce to put on top by mixing the chopped tomatoes with tomato purée.

■ Have fun preparing the toppings together. Grate the cheese, and slice the sausages, ham, mushrooms and peppers.

■ Ask your child to choose what to put on the top of the pizzas, finishing with the grated cheese. Encourage your child to think of his/her own ideas such as creating 'funny faces'.

■ Put the pizzas under the grill until the cheese is bubbling. Leave to cool slightly before eating.

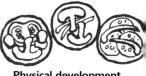

# Maisy moves house

One day Maisy's dad told her some exciting news.

'Maisy,' said Dad, 'Mum and I have decided to build our own house.'

Maisy's dad was a builder and her mum was a plumber, so they were going to build most of the house themselves. They took Maisy in the builder's van to see the big piece of land where the house was going to be built.

'This is our plot,' they said and they all ran around it with excitement.

'This is where the kitchen will be,' smiled Mum, jumping up and down.

'And here is the front door,' laughed Dad, waving his hands in the air.

'Don't forget my bedroom,' shouted Maisy, pointing upwards.

Mum and Dad swung Maisy up in the air.

'Hooray for the new house!' giggled Maisy. 'When I grow up I'm going to be a builder like you, Dad'.

'Good, because I've got a surprise for you,' whispered Dad into Maisy's ear. 'Come over here'. He carried Maisy to a corner of the building plot. 'This is your very own building plot! Mum and I are going to help you to build your own little house here. It will only be big enough for you and your friends, no grown-ups'.

'I'm going to be a builder, I'm going to be a builder,' chanted Maisy happily.

Mum and Dad worked hard on the family house over the next few months and showed Maisy how to put the bricks in rows to make the walls of her little house. As they fitted the doors and windows, they showed Maisy how to do the same. When the roof was put on the big house, a tiny roof was put on to Maisy's house.

Once the big house was finished, Mum and Dad chose the wallpaper and paint while Maisy chose some for the inside of her little house.

At last the big removal vans came to Maisy's old house to carry all of their things to the new houses.

'Party time!' said Mum, and invited all of their friends to a barbecue in the garden. At the same time Maisy had her own house-warming tea party in the little house with her special friends, Rosie and George.

'Thank you for showing me how to build a house, Mum and Dad', said Maisy. 'I can't wait to grow up and start work!'.

Jean Evans

# Secret places

When we help to unpack the shopping
Me and my brother Ben,
We pile up the boxes and packets
To make a super den.

When we help to bring in washing
Me and my brother Ben,
We hang the towels over the chairs
To make a secret den.

When we give the dog his dinner
Me and my brother Ben,
We scramble into his kennel
To share his special den.

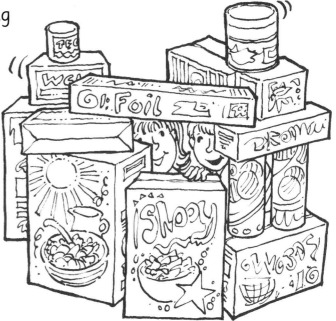

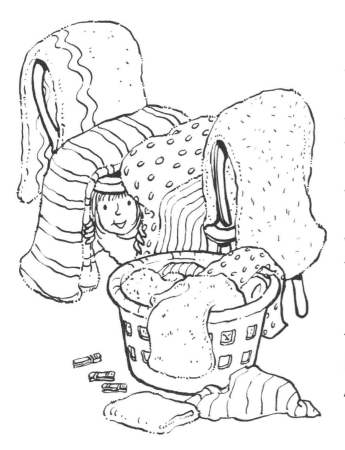

When we help to draw the curtains
Me and my brother Ben,
We hide behind the frills and folds
To make a floaty den.

When we go upstairs at bedtime,
Me and my brother Ben,
We bury under the bedclothes
To make a cosy den.

Dens are dark and exciting places
To hide yourself away,
Do you make dens around your house
As secret places to play?

Jean Evans

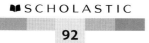

# Ahoy there!

*Tune: 'This Old Man'*

Riding over the ocean blue
The captain and his pirate crew
And 'Ahoy there, Ahoy there,' we hear them loudly cry,
As their ship goes sailing by.

Hoisting the flag, up the mast,
The Jolly Roger is fluttering past,
And 'Ahoy there, Ahoy there,' we hear them loudly cry,
As their ship goes sailing by.

Up and down through the waves,
To land on shores with deep dark caves,
And 'Ahoy there, Ahoy there,' we hear them loudly cry,
As their ship goes sailing by.

Looking for treasure the pirate band,
Will dig their holes along the sand,
And 'Ahoy there, Ahoy there,' we hear them loudly cry,
As their ship goes sailing by.

Searching East, searching West,
For gold to fill a treasure chest,
And 'Ahoy there, Ahoy there,' we hear them loudly cry,
As their ship goes sailing by.

Jean Evans

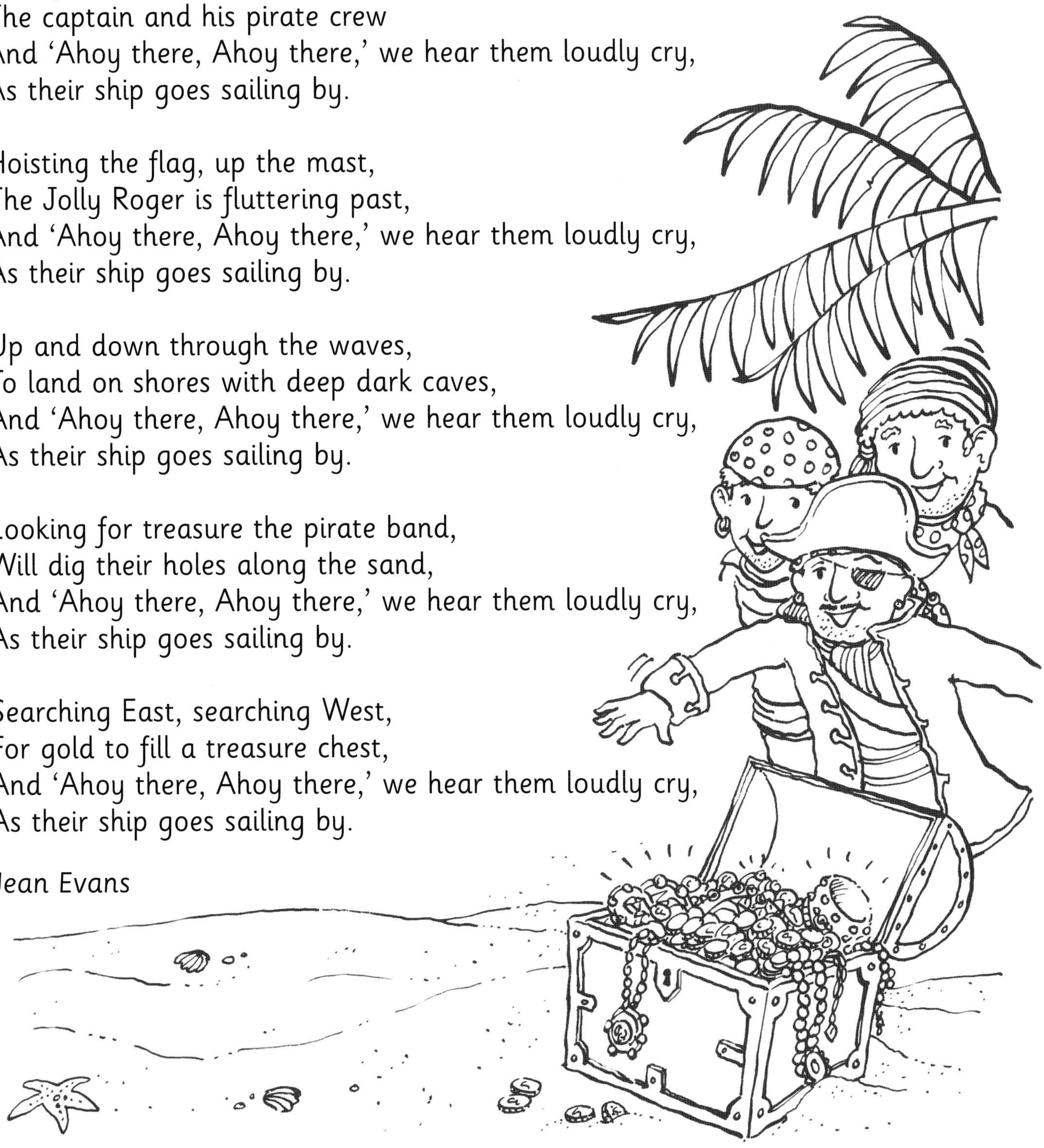

**SCHOLASTIC**

# Odd one out

Put a large cross through the odd sock and colour in the matching two socks.

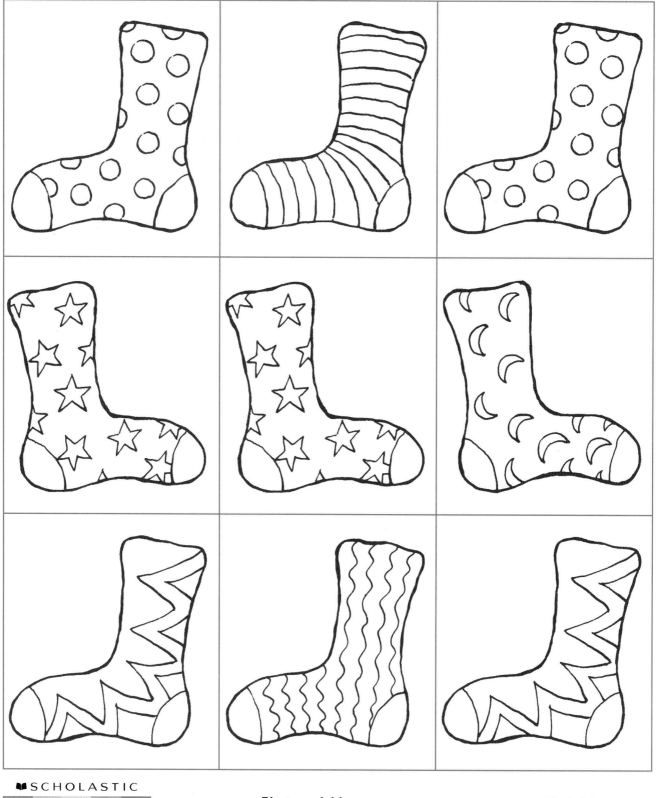

**Photocopiable**

**Physical development**

# Play-dough recipe

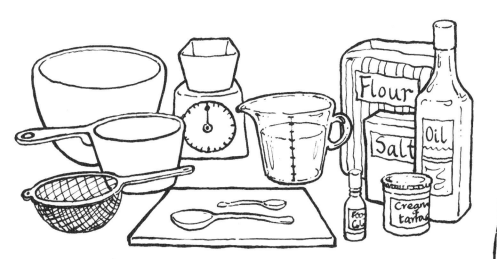

## What to do

◼ Weigh out 200g of plain flour and 100g of salt, then to measure two teaspoons of cream of tartar and one tablespoon of cooking oil.

◼ Put all the ingredients into the saucepan.

◼ Measure 300ml of water in a jug and add a few drops of food colouring to it before pouring it gently into the pan.

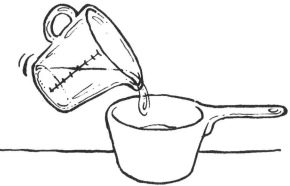

◼ Stir the mixture well.

◼ Heat the mixture slowly until it forms a stiff ball.

◼ Tip the play dough on to a pastry board and leave it to cool.

◼ When the dough is cool, let your child play with it. Encourage him/her to try patting, stroking, poking, squeezing, pinching and twisting it.

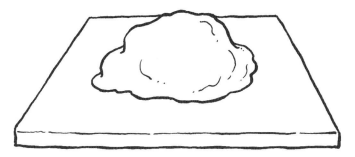

# The Divali story

Once, long ago in India, a king had a son, the prince Rama. The prince wanted to marry the beautiful princess, Sita, so he decided to visit her. Sita's father said to him, 'See if you are strong enough to lift up my heavy bow and bend it.'

Rama lifted up the bow and bent it until it broke into pieces.

'I can see that you are very strong, so you can marry Sita,' said her father.

Rama and Sita got married and Rama took his new wife to meet his father, the king.

One day the old king said, 'When I die I want Rama to be the new king.' But the queen wanted Rama's brother, Prince Bharat, to be king.

'Send Rama away,' she said.

The king was sad but he sent Rama away for fourteen years. Rama went into the forest with Sita and her brother, Lakshman.

When the king died, the queen told Prince Bharat that he could be king, but the prince remembered that his father wanted Rama to be king.

'No,' he said, 'I must go and get Rama.'

He searched the forest to find Rama, Sita and Lakshman.

'Come back home, Rama,' he said. 'You should be the new king now.'

'But I promised I would stay away for fourteen years,' said Rama.

'Then give me your golden sandals,' said Prince Bharat.

He put Rama's sandals on the old king's throne and told the people, 'Rama is the new king but until he comes back I will look after you.'

Rama and Sita stayed in the forest. One day a wicked demon called Ravana, with ten arms and ten heads, captured Sita and locked her in his castle on a faraway island.

'I want to marry you, Sita,' said Ravana.

'No,' said Sita, firmly.

Rama and Lakshman searched for Sita everywhere until Hanuman, the king of the monkeys, told them where she was. His monkeys built a strong bridge so that Rama and his friends could cross the sea to Ravana's castle. In a big fight, Rama killed Ravana with a magic arrow and rescued Sita.

'Fourteen years have now past, Sita,' said Rama. 'We can go home again.'

They travelled home on an elephant's back. It was very dark when they arrived so the people put little lights called divas outside their houses to help them to find the way. Everyone was happy because Rama was home again.

Retold by Jean Evans

Photocopiable

Physical development